BIRTH AND OTHER SURPRISES

PRAISE FOR KIMBERLY DAVIS BASSO

"Roll on the floor hilarity"

— NEIL WHITE, AUTHOR OF TURN A BLIND EYE

"A wicked, wicked sense of humor. I'd like to meet her."

— CATH AND KINDLE REVIEWS

"All the flair of a standup comedian [Basso] reminds me why I like talented writers so much."

— WRITER'S DIGEST, JUDGES NOTES

"Wildly honest, heartbreakingly human."

— TANIA KATAN, AUTHOR OF MY ONE NIGHT STAND WITH CANCER

"We are held by fear. We are held by laughter. Oh how well Basso wields this double-edged sword."

— JULIA SIMPSON URRUTIA, AUTHOR OF THE RED SEA BRIDE

Early Praise for Birth and Other Surprises

"Basso makes you laugh, makes you laugh loud and hard as you move through the ridiculous, the sublime... It's only after that you realize what she's done, that through her humor she brings you deeper into the great truth, that is Basso's gift."

— WILLIAM QUIGLEY AUTHOR OF JOY BLISS THIS

"After reading Basso's book on childbirth, I will never look at the chest burster scene in *Alien* the same way."

— BRADLEY UPTON, AUTHOR OF BLOOD STAKES

BIRTH AND OTHER SURPRISES

KIMBERLY DAVIS BASSO

INGRAMSPARK

First printing, 2020

Print ISBN 978-1-7345523-0-0

Ebook ISBN 978-1-7345523-1-7

Cover Lettering by Amanda Crevier www.AmandaCrevier.ca

Author Photo by Donna Alberico, www.DonnaAlberico.com

To my uterus-

Well done.

CONTENTS

BEGIN

Defined: *verb* To come into existence, arrive.

You have to start somewhere.

NAILED THE LANDING

I wasn't born, I arrived.

YES, I was delivered by aliens. Deposited me in a lovely field of grass, surrounded by beautiful trees. Or so I was told. The alien part, not the trees and meadow part, that's what I assumed. In reality, if aliens delivered me it was in a smoking, rusty canister that crash landed in our backyard, which my parents finally noticed when my brother woke the neighborhood by whacking it with a baseball bat. Canister and contents unceremoniously dropped at the town dump on Saturday—end of story. Not that I've thought about it or anything.

In truth we were driving home from our weekly visit to my grandmother's house, and my dad took a different route. Being the youngest I was required to sit, knees hunched on the hump in the middle, peering at the tops of the trees out the car window. But these were the wrong trees.

"Where are we going?"

"We're taking you back to the field where we found you. Where the aliens dropped you off," said my brother.

"Cool."

I settled back to see this field of destiny for myself. Not the slightest concern, not a care in the world. Unfortunately, my dad was only trying one of his many shortcuts. We still haven't gotten home.

In all likelihood I was born. As far as I know. I mean, I was there, but I can't honestly remember a thing. I assume it's like this for everyone. Everyone except the current generation, who will be able to watch their own in-vitro videos, to be topped only by the following generation, who will have in utero Go Pros™ to record their special journey down the birth canal:

"And on your left – moms ovaries!!! On your right, behind the condom that broke and got stuck behind a fallopian tube – a rest stop for other eggs and a short order cook making them snacks!"

That's physically impossible, by the way, just in case you're one of many adults these days who seem to need a lesson in female anatomy. The short order cook always hangs out near the labia.

The current story is that I was delivered not by aliens, but by a nurse because my doctor was still in the parking lot. It happens. When a woman shows up at the hospital at 5:43 pm and the kid is born before 6 pm, there's a chance a few people will miss it. Dad missed it but that was planned, because back then men weren't allowed to see their wives' vaginas give birth. Too delicate to handle the shock that what they put in was going to come back out, rip roaring and rarin' to go. I'm sure it came as a great surprise to me as well, though I don't recall exactly what I had planned that day. I assume I had some laps to do, couple of flip turns. Soccer practice. Maybe just a good stretch and a nap but apparently arriving was on the agenda. Upon meeting me, my brother and sister took off everything but my diaper and counted my fingers and toes. Seems there was early suspicion about my alien status.

Yes, everyone has a birth story and yours is the most interesting. But since none of us have been what you'd call 'present' at our own births, or at least, aware enough to discuss it later, the birth story that matters is the one we can tell. The birth of our child. Everyone has a story. Every. One. And each one is the best birth story. The birth story is the moment that you became a parent – it might be in a delivery room, it might be in a court room, it might be with a child who is older or not born yet, doesn't matter – it's the moment that your heart unlocks and the key is lost forever, opening a floodgate. A floodgate of love and a huge slimy backwash of judgment from other people, most of them strangers.

Given that everyone's birth story is awesome and the only one you really care about is yours, let's discuss why we're here. Perhaps you're reading this book to pass the time between finding out you were pregnant and giving birth. Forty weeks is a long time. Or, you're reading this book because you're a parent and you'd like to feel better about the job you're doing. You're killing it! Go ahead and compare yourself to me, happy to help inflate your ego at no extra charge. I'm certain you're doing a better job than I am. Just ask my kids. And that guy in the grocery store who insisted I give my toddler candy because she was having a fit. By all means, sugar up the angry kid.

We'll also discuss some medical procedures, because unlike other medical procedures, birth is not a medical procedure. Unlike medical procedures, birth requires neither medicine nor procedure. We proceed medically anyway, just to be safe, but it differs greatly in this regard from say, a sliced artery. Or an exploding appendix. The "patient" or "baby" is simply arriving. Like a spaceship. Or a passenger jet. Hopefully a very small one. Presumably there have been no intervening medical procedures since inception, those being extremely rare and also freaking amazing. In utero surgery? Are you kidding? That's a thing we can do? We can fix a problem in the baby's heart before arrival? Astonishing. That would be like someone finding your luggage and correctly re-routing it before you knew it was missing. Sounds impossible – but how would you know?

Likewise, I won't know if you read this book out of order, in fact, I encourage you to flip around to parts that sound interesting. It's excellent preparation for the non-linear art of parenting and the years of multi-tasking involved. See Parenting Work Flow below for details or just put this book down at random moments, lose it for weeks on end, discover it under the couch (or possibly as part of a permanent "fort" exhibit in the hallway) and then attempt to pick up where you left off. Let several birthdays pass in between. Sufficiently confused? Our preparations are working already.

CHART: Parenting Work Flow

We regret to inform you that the chart Parenting Work Flow *is unavailable. We fed the parent multi-tasking data into one of those super computers, a really good one, like the kind that can play chess, calculate asteroid disasters and create recipes for brownies that have nothing but the chewy edges all at the same time. The result was a high-pitched whine. For a fun home craft representation of Parenting Work Flow, overcook a bowl of spaghetti three different ways and then throw it on the floor. It won't precisely replicate the complexity of parenting, but you may as well get used to abusing dinner and having crap lying around.*

FORGING AHEAD TO A SYNOPSIS. Why a synopsis, you ask? Well, the baby could come at any time, right? Right. No, I mean that. Let's repeat it. The baby could come at any time. I feel like you aren't understanding the emphasis here. The baby could come at **any** time.

Any time. Like before you reach the end of this page. Or this sentence. If you understand nothing else about birth, understand this – it doesn't matter how much you prepared, it doesn't matter how you want it to go, it doesn't matter what your plans are. There is no act of will strong enough to deny your baby the entrance into the world that s/he is going to have. And this is the crux of the problem – as adults we assume that preparing for something means you are having an impact on the result. You are not. Should you still prepare? Yes, because it sucks to be at the hospital without the comfy toilet paper. Do not assume that you will control this. It could all go according to your fondest birth plan wishes and I sincerely hope it does. And it could all go completely sideways. Either way – it's not because of something you did. No, really. There's another human involved in the birth of your child, namely the child – and they have not read your birth plan. They are not interested in your birth plan. I'm sure it's a nice plan, I'm sure it has some great ideas and some interesting ideas and some that are just straight up wacko in your own 'you gotta be you' way and it required a lot of forethought and good for you. Doesn't matter. My suggestion is this:

Make a plan. Prepare in whatever ways make you feel most comfortable and give you the most pleasure in your pregnancy. Take care of yourself in the healthiest way possible for you. Imagine how you'd like it all to happen. And know that you've just strapped yourself into a rollercoaster, and not only has this particular roller coaster never been ridden, no one actually knows where it goes. Screaming may very well be, you know, totally appropriate. Giving birth is in fact, the perfect preamble to parenting in that way. Well done Mother Nature.

TIME

Defined: A limited period or interval. Labor does not obey this law. On time: dependable, prompt, reliable, punctual, timely, without delay, on schedule. Not late. Or as we say in our house, "other people." Related phrases: "Ahead of time" a phrase you'll likely never use again.

Antonyms: Late. But since you're going to be experiencing this a lot, here are some options: missed the boat (nautically minded); held up (criminally minded); postponed (optimistic); overdue (bookish); tardy (educators); belated (birthday wishes only, please); unpunctual (which seems ungrammatical); lagging (nice over tone of depression); eleventh hour (the name of my late night talk show); and my personal favorite: behindhand. As in "I do everything behindhand."

PRECISION AND THE ART OF PREGNANCY

My husband and I are the same vintage. Born just before the seventies got rolling, just in time for truly atrocious fashion and the last slow era of childhood. Summer lasted most of the year and school was an occasional event. Memories can be delicious, can't they? I've been accused of being obsessed with time, and nothing exacerbates my illness like parenting. It seems best to address this here near the start. As a parent to be you are now entered in a time vortex. Time will be sliced in numerous ways, the most absurd of which is the forty-week timeline of pregnancy. We won't go into time as a construct, or how in reality it can be sliced however you'd like it to be. That's for Einstein and his newer, hipper counterpart Neil deGrasse Tyson to figure out.

Remember that parenting flow chart that blew up the computers? It starts with the first time you are asked, "So, when are you having kids?" The moment Lovely Boyfriend and I became Lovely Hubby and I we were asked if we were making plans to make babies. While it's interesting that other people have time to consider the factory like uses of my uterus, it's not really, oh, what's the word, anybody's business. I won't pretend here to know or care when or if you should have kids, or more kids, or one kid, or ten kids. Or if your kids should be planned or spontaneous or spontaneously combust (hopefully not this last, I live in Southern California, and you know, wildfires).

Instead, let's tackle something simple to start; going on a trip with children. One details of note, I did not in fact say a 'vacation.' I said a 'trip with children.' Don't panic, it boils down to this:

Remember to bring the kids. Yes, all of them.

I know. So easy. You think it's absurd to bring this up so early in our discussion. Or perhaps you think 'remember to bring the kids' is unworthy of any mention at all. Do you know why no one else talks about this? Because it didn't happen to them. It happened to me. I was left behind in my crib when my family went on vacation. And I wasn't even talking yet so it's not like I was annoying them in an overwhelming way. They packed the car, packed the stuff, packed the kids, drove away.

I don't think they got far. Maybe a mile up the road? My siblings probably weren't arguing yet because when my brother asked, "Where's the baby?" they could actually hear him.

They turned the car around, got the baby, packed the car, packed the stuff, packed the kids, packed the baby, drove away. I can't imagine what they concocted to cover this blunder. Or if they bothered to – people in the seventies didn't feel the need to be perfect all the time. After all, there was no one recording anything. If we took pictures, we may or may not have remembered to develop the film after the vacation. Sometimes it melted before it was developed because it was left in the trunk along with the keys for four hours while we stood in that really hot parking lot. See? I have no idea where that trip was, but the experience stayed with me because my parents remembered to bring me along.

I'm not alone in this, it also happened to Lovely Hubby. His family left him behind at a restaurant while he was waiting for a stranger to finish drinking a beer so he could have the can for his collection. Kids can be so creative.

I do wonder though, if this early abandonment while the family fled the scene led to my concerns over time. I am extremely antsy when I'm needed to be on time somewhere. As noted in that other book, trying to be on time for heart surgery nearly killed me. But it isn't just the huge medical issues. It's the day by day, 'how many appointments do I have today' running clock in my head which barely compares to the gigantic question, when will the baby arrive? If you've been paying attention, you know the real answer is any damn time the baby wants to. Nevertheless, we try and hold them to an appointment. That's a lot of pressure to put on a new human, and on a mother-to-be frankly. Regardless of where the baby is exiting (your own uterus or someone else's), arrival times are important. And the closer you get to the day, the tighter the tension grows. Multiply anything in this book by a million for the first baby. Two million if it's the first grandchild on either side.

The due date. The date your human being is due. It just seems unfair to lock them into a specific twenty-four hours after a ten-month journey. Most people can't meet for coffee on schedule. Airlines can't get us from here to there in the three hours they promised it would take. And have you ever met a single doctor who could actually meet with patients at the appointed time? And yet we all accept it and expect it of the new arrival. An overdue baby? How dare they! Clearly there's a problem. I'd like to see some monitors in the waiting room on the maternity floor, just like in an airport. All the mom-to-be stats up there. A nice graphic over to the right showing relative size of the vaginal opening throughout dilation. Nurses could work a little betting action on the side. Here's my question: Why is the baby capable of handling forty weeks of development on its own, but is considered unqualified to make its own entrance?

For forty weeks, little whomever swims along, developing this, creating that, adding in the little bits and bobs that make up a human.

Kicking moving squirming doing all the fun in utero yoga that goes on. And then, suddenly a panic – how can this helpless creature possibly know when it's ready to arrive? It seems a bit odd, doesn't it? It's a due date. The baby is due on this date and if it's not there it's overdue. Like a library book. Speaking of, did you know libraries are free? For you. Not us. My family is happily underwriting our library and probably several others with our overdue fees. Now there's a thought! Charge the baby! Charge the baby for being late. If you're any kind of a decent parent you already have them enrolled in college, right? So just add it to the debt. Boom. Solved.

Turns out it wasn't always this way. It's only relatively recently that giving birth became a medical event. In the mid 1700's the first school for midwives was opened by a gentleman named Who Cares because read that again. In the mid 1700's a gentleman opened a school for midwives. A gentleman. So roughly thousands of years after our species arrived and the whole birth thing was a huge success, the human population running rampant over the planet, a dude decides to teach women how to help other women give birth. Sure Kimberly, why not? After all, men at that time were well versed in the workings of the female body, seeing as they spent no time studying the female body. Lot of guess work happening. Still happening.

To no one's surprise, many midwives didn't bother to attend the "dude teaches you how to do what you already know" seminar. Probably too busy helping women give birth. Also not a shock – the first people to adopt the new practices, i.e., "a male doctor in a hospital setting" were wealthy, because only someone with money to spare would be able to have a doctor help. Don't get me wrong – it's important to have medical care, and no one is suggesting you birth to your kid on a rooftop assisted by an orangutan and an orange. Though I hear that's a movement. But I do find it odd that we are taking a stopwatch to something that for millennia just… happened. Then again, a baby alien is about to invade your life, so maybe hold onto that due date. Maybe hold onto that due date like it's the Holy Grail and you are the last in the line of Templar Knights. That due date is a piece of specific information, a life raft in a world of uncertainty. Go for it. Whatever makes you feel good. Fortunately, treating the baby like a library book is starting to shift, and the actual size of the baby is used to determine how many weeks have gone by and when arrival is likely. Which of course, leads to the absurd obsession with age and size that lingers until they are two. I mean twenty-four months.

Where did the whole forty weeks on the dot thing come from? A scientist. With a penis. The standard rule is to add a year from a woman's last period, subtract three months and add a week because math is fun. Gets you to two hundred and eighty days, or exactly ten cycles long. If, and only if, your cycle is exactly twenty-eight days long and you ovulate exactly halfway at fourteen days and you got pregnant at the exact halfway point of your fertile time. It's all very sexy no? Oui. I don't know about you, but my eggs are not that organized. They line up in the carton but once we start cooking all bets are off. The cookie cutter approach just doesn't cut it and frankly it's an awful lot of pressure to put on an alien. Baby. It's an awful lot of pressure to put on a baby to arrive on that day. You think you could build a machine that complex, and have it done on time? Ever had a kitchen renovated? I promise, not a chance of that happening. It would be fine to calculate based on a formula, if in fact you have a different formula for every woman. Individualized care, the hallmark of the entire medical system. Sorry, this is supposed to be non-fiction.

The due date, the deadline of all deadlines. The one piece of information that every expectant parent knows. You may or may not know the gender of your child to be, you may or may not know what the name will be, you may or may not know who the biological father is, but you for damn sure know when it is supposed to exit your uterus.

A SIMPLE REQUEST

The following letter was found crumpled on the floor near a weeping mom desperately trying to jam her three month old's foot into a onesie marked "twelve months" after she gave up trying to put him in one marked "newborn" because it was so huge it fell off when she picked him up.

DEAR BABY STUFF COMPANY:

Why months?

Why is everything measured in months? Why do you insist on labeling baby clothes on a monthly system, as if the time you spend on the planet is somehow directly related to how big or small you are? I appreciate being served time in small manageable increments less likely to induce panic as we realize she's one hundred and fifty-six months and is getting her driver's license in... wait... I need a minute to do the math...

Sure, it's fun to watch this bizarre system confuse the hell out of friends without kids. But I devised my own way to torture my friends, thank you, it's called "can you babysit for just an hour or so?" The monthly, leftover counting from pregnancy size label thing is just weird. Particularly since there do not seem to be any rules regarding, say, the length of a onesie and its label as "newborn" or "six months." I humbly suggest a new labeling system, closer to what actually occurs:

•Brand Spanking New and May or May Not Be Smallish

•Medium-er, Not as Shiny, Probably has Some Boogers

•Noticeably Bigger but Still Not Sleeping the Night

•Who is this Giant Child and Why is She Borrowing My Clothes?

•Just Because You're Taller than I am Doesn't Mean – You Come Back Here Right Now!

Thanks!

Mama Bear

P.S. If you'd like to confuse and educate at the same time, use fractions.

P.P.S. Thanks ever so much for encasing absolutely everything in plastic so you have somewhere to print that "plastic bags aren't toys" warning.

EGG AND SPERM MEET CUTE

A SHORT FILM

Cast: One Egg, 500 bazillion Sperm

BACKSTORY:

Remarkably, one sperm out of thousands penetrates the egg. One. Out of thousands. I can only assume the rate is that high because the sperm does not have to interact or ask permission. It's odd that the end result of sex is so unsexy. At least, that's what I keep drilling into my someday to be teenagers children. Think about it. Imagine the pickup lines, if they were honest:

"Hi, I'd like to have sex with you, and no matter what we do, the potential end result (beer belch) is that we'd make a person who poops in their pants."

ENOUGH OF THAT. ACTION!

Fade up on Sperm, followed by 499 bazillion identical brothers, as he approaches Egg, lounging comfortably in the uterine wall (just CGI it, there's no way you can build something that complex, and if you can, the entire female population would love to see it).

Sperm: Hello, I'm Sperm and these are thousands of my identical brothers.

Egg: Hi.

Sperm: Yeah, I'm the representative, but – back off Charlie – any one of us, any one of us, is just dying to burrow through and make a connection. So, what do you say?

Egg: Uh, well I like the connection part. How do I choose?

Sperm: Choose? Oh, you don't get to choose. We're all going to swarm you at once.

Egg: What do you mean you're all going to swarm at once? How is that possible?

Sperm: Well, some of us will get kicked in the head, or rather, whipped by a tail to the head, but still, it's everybody, all at one time.

Egg: Couldn't I, say, do some interviews? Or at least pick my top fifty? Thousands seems like a lot. There's bound to be some assholes in there. Just from a statistical point of view.

Sperm: Nope. It's all or nothing.

Egg: Well, OK. But this better work. You guys swarm all over me and nothing comes of it, I'm going to just crumple up and fade away, you got that?

Sperm: Yes, ma'am. This is a one shot deal for us too.

Egg: OK. Good luck.

Decidedly unsexy music swells as we fade to black.

BIRDS AND BEES AND PUPPIES

At some point, some type of conversation about sex will happen with your child, so fill it with excellent information and delightful diagrams. Or you can get existential and return the question, "Where did any of us come from? Why are we here? And more importantly, why is the cat in the dresser drawer?" My parents opted for a less conventional model using pets, our family dogs Pride and Joy. That's right, Pride and Joy. Because what my parents really wanted was a boat. Pride and Joy were beagles and they had all the delightful beagle traits like yapping, running, yapping, chasing after rabbits, yapping, hunting, running, stealing things from the neighbors' BBQ. Yes, that was us. That time that an entire package of hotdogs disappeared, and then a few minutes later, a package of rolls? Yes, that was our dog. Dad thought it was funny to send her back for the rolls. Oh, and beagles? They yap all day, among other things. When the dog run is next to a giant bush that is home base for a family of rabbits, well, nature happens. Luckily I was too young to fully understand what the brown fluffs of fur strewn all over the back yard meant.

Our two yappers were purebred beagles, and they did what any male and female animals of age do – they made more. I was four years old and all I knew was that Joy was going to have puppies. Very exciting. No idea what it meant. I woke up on New Year's Day and there were seven little puppies downstairs with her, and her husband, as I thought of him, had been banished. Summarily dismissed, without a backward glance. Looking back, I don't know if that was a 'protect the pups from everyone' maneuver or a 'look what you got me into you bastard' maneuver, but either way, he was not allowed near her. And to be safe, neither were we. No need to rile Mama. But my parents did want to have her checked, so they went off to the vet. Yes, I grew up in a time that the vet would meet you at the office on a holiday because your dog had puppies and you wanted to make sure she was OK. Don't get excited, the seventies weren't all rainbows and glitter (see the chapter on safety for more). It was also a time that the vet would examine your dog and kindly inform you, "You better get her out of here, she's going to have another puppy, and if she does I have to charge you for delivering it."

Back at home with the first seven puppies, we were oblivious. No idea of the impending additional arrival, because my Dad and brother went to the vet, and mom stayed home to call around to let everyone know. In the seventies, only one person could be called at a time, and there was no group texting or chatting. Or even faxing for that matter. Occasionally dinosaurs would carry messages for us but only if we asked nicely.

Mom was on call nineteen, "Oh, yes, Joy had seven puppies. Seven! I know, she did so well. Gotta go, lots of calls to..."

In runs dad from the vet, "Eight puppies! She had another on the drive back."

Yes, he had to drive all the way home and run into the kitchen before he could tell her that our dog birthed another puppy in the car, because the phone was physically attached to the wall by what we called a "cord." Mom laughed and started calling everyone back, until he runs two minutes later:

"Make it nine puppies, just delivered another one in the car in the driveway."

And then the soundtrack for *101 Dalmatians*™ started…Wow. Nine puppies out of that tiny body. That's a double litter, if not triple, for a beagle, I assume, because she ran out of nipples. You read that correctly. She had more puppies than nipples to feed them with. Seems like poor engineering. No wonder she wanted her mate dead. My mom had to rotate the puppies as they ate, just to make sure they got food. I can only assume this is what people with triplets do. Kids gotta eat!

Joy did get over her anger or her instincts and we were finally allowed to play with the pups. She had no choice really, as we had to help her feed them. I defy you to give a four-year-old more fun than lying down on the floor and having nine puppies crawl all over her. Don't bother, it can't be done. It was absolutely delightful. Tiny little soft claws on even softer paw pads. They stepped on my stomach, my face, they got caught in my hair. I laughed for three days straight. I distinctly remember helping my mom put together some kind of liquid food for them, I assume now to help Joy keep up with feeding her family. Around the same time, my mother and I got horribly sick, and yet, it was still Mom's job to help feed the pups. I'm not sure why that's true, but it was. Maybe it was just that they needed round the clock feeding, but I recall my mom crawling downstairs with peanut butter covers full of some sort of milk substance for the puppies. At four years old I had my first two examples of moms getting the job done regardless of reality (not enough nipples) or their own health (what was probably influenza). What stayed with me, of course, was not the lesson; in fact, it only just occurred to me that this was a distinctly mom moment. All I remember were soft little faces and tiny ears rubbing against my cheek, noses snuffling in my hair.

I had no way of knowing at the time that my parents were using the puppies as sex education for my brother and sister, who were somewhere in the nine years old range. Having a birth (or nine) happen in the house is as good a way to teach about reproduction as any, and certainly better than say the mold spores growing in that leftover food bin in the fridge. Alas, I was too young, so I learned on New Year's Eve that the puppies were going to arrive at some point in the future and then boom – there they were on New Year's Day. I was certainly disappointed that my own pregnancies took quite a bit longer.

My personal intro to sex education, at least, what I learned from my family, was conducted as my mother and I walked to my dance class a mile away. Correction, it wasn't sex education, because we were Catholic. We didn't have sex, we procreated. And it was made very clear that sex or anything like it would not be happening until I was married, or the world would end and then right after the world ended my parents would kill me. That's a fairly succinct message with little room for misinterpretation. Sex leads to death. Got it. Given my response, they needn't have worried. At least not at that point. I can't imagine my mom bringing up the subject, and it only took about twelve words start to finish. You'll forgive me that I don't have the pre-amble recorded here, but the rest is verbatim:

"The man puts his penis into the woman's..."

Pause

"Into it? Actually into it?"

"Yes."

"Ew."

And that was it. The sum total of information I officially received from my parents. I was ten, maybe eleven, I believe. Given our religious status, I understand why. And I can't see my parents have a conversation with me about this – they are of a generation that simply did not discuss, so I'm probably lucky I got that much info. I do realize how fortunate I was to have the kind of friends I did, and the kind of boyfriends I did, because I know plenty of people whose Sex

Ed was left up to the general population. Which tends to add to the general population. Strange, isn't it? The less you know about how sex works, the more likely you are to create a baby. Of course, you can always tell your kids they were delivered by aliens and hope for the best. It won't work, but you can do it.

HOW TO GROW A BABY

Apologies for not mentioning this earlier – there are things that you don't have to worry about, like how to grow a baby. And thank goodness, because the marketing would be weird. Remember those strange little critters they used to advertise in the back of comic books? Some sort of Mer-people wearing crowns so you could "Grow Your Own Underwater Kingdom"? I'm pretty sure they were just shrimp. Maybe some kind of bug. I never quite achieved a kingdom. Or queendom for that matter. Just a smelly cup of brine water.

Seriously, this is the absolute best part about growing a baby: do nothing. Once you've decided that there is going to be a baby— either before during or after the sperm and the egg connect successfully— there's not a lot to do except not take up heroin. Your body already knows everything. And I mean everything. Which is a huge relief. Can you imagine if you had to grow each part of your baby personally? Like, not just every finger and toe, but every nerve ending? Every organ? Every skin cell? It's impossible, it's a master work of engineering there simply is no comparison. We can ooh and ahh all we want about the great and amazing things that humanity has constructed over the years, but it don't mean diddly next to humanity itself. Even with all the advances in science, all the ways that fertilization can be supported, once fertilized, that fetus is off and running and even then, things don't always coalesce because it is just so damn complex. An astonishing feat of engineering. I can barely handle a Lego™ set with more than thirty pieces. I think of all the plants I've killed over the years and I know I would not be right for that job. Thank you, Mother Nature.

HOW TO GROW A PARENT

Ah, this is entirely different from growing a baby. There are so very many ways to go about this and yet they all end up in the same place— you + a kid = parent. Shocking that it's as simple as that. Given the implications of raising a human, you'd think there'd be more to it. Nope. The kid is yours. Maybe you were directly involved in the biology, maybe you weren't. Doesn't matter. You have a kid? You're a parent. It may seem odd to stress this, but I've recently been in the school parking lot and you'd be surprised how many people seem surprised by the existence of their own progeny. They're rushing through the drop off lane like it's an Indy 500 pit stop and they just can't wait to leave. Fine, but please make sure Johnny is actually fully out of the car before you hit the gas.

When I was in utero, no one read parenting books. "Parent," in fact, was a noun, not a verb. I recall sitting in church one day, not when I was in utero mind you, much later, and for who knows what reason the sermon was about parenting books. The priest told a joke about new parents frantically flipping through a book while their child cried, and the punch line of course was "put down the book, pick up the child." Everyone laughed and felt excellent about themselves. Still, given how much we know now about how little we knew then (baby powder anyone?) a little research might not be a bad idea. You could prepare by reading serious books on the subject (and there are thousands). You could prepare by reading not so serious books on the subject (thank you). You could try a birthing class, if the new human is entering the world from your body, or the body of someone you know. Lots of choices there. There's natural childbirth, hypnobirth, water birth, birthing while on horseback, birthing while doing your taxes, birthing while at work, in the bathroom, in an ambulance, on the moon. Take your pick. There are even sibling birthing class options – how to be jealous, how to act like you aren't jealous so everyone thinks you're amazing, how to out-cute the baby (impossible, don't waste your money), how to hug the baby without looking like you're trying to strangle it. That kind of thing.

Here's the good news – you get to grow, with your child. Kind of the way your body does in pregnancy, though hopefully not as awkwardly. Was it just me, or did the shift in your gravitational center also affect the tides? You won't be starting off with a teenager, or heaven forbid, a pre-teenager. You'll get a baby. The list of needs is short and simple, and nearly impossible to fulfill without exhaustion. If you are able to fulfill it without exhaustion be a dear and don't tell anyone. We don't want to know. We mostly think 1) you're lying or 2) you have a nanny to do the heavy lifting 3) you're some kind of saint. Whatever it is, don't tell us. We still want to be friends with you and we're not sure we can carry that kind of resentment and still keep this relationship going. Where were we? Ah, yes, growing with your child.

The list before the baby is born can be overwhelming if you let it. So much stuff! George Carlin would be proud. Once the baby is born, the list becomes very straightforward:

Did the baby Eat? Burp? Sleep? Pee? Poop?

Eat? Burp? Sleep? Pee? Poop?

Eat? Burp? Sleep? Pee? Poop? Eat? Burp? Sleep? Pee? Poop?

Eat? Burp? Sleep? Pee? Poop? Eat? Burp? Sleep? Pee? Poop? Eat? Burp? Sleep? Pee? Poop? Eat? Burp? Sleep? Pee? Poop? Eat? Burp? Sleep? Pee? Poop? Eat? Burp? Sleep? Pee? Poop? Eat? Burp? Sleep? Pee? Poop? Eat? Burp? Sleep? Pee? Poop? Eat? Burp? Sleep? Pee? Poop? Eat? Burp? Sleep? Pee? Poop? Eat? Burp? Sleep? Pee? Poop? Eat? Burp? Sleep? Pee? Poop? Eat? Burp? Sleep? Pee? Poop? Eat? Burp? Sleep? Pee? Poop? Eat? Burp? Sleep? Pee? Poop? Eat? Burp? Sleep? Pee? Poop? Eat? Burp? Sleep? Pee? Poop?Eat? Burp? Sleep? Pee? Poop? Eat? Burp? Sleep? Pee? Poop? Eat? Burp? Sleep? Pee? Poop? Eat? Burp? Sleep? Pee? Poop?

Incredibly, it is possible to forget one of these. My child was crying inconsolably at the age of eighteen hours and I couldn't figure out why. Got as far as Eat, Burp, Sleep on the list and forgot the rest. She was stuck in that loop with me, utterly miserable. Turns out she had a gallon and a half of pee in her diaper. Well, that would make anyone cranky. The needs are not difficult to handle, just difficult to remember when sleep deprived. Oh, yes. That little list of needs is an around the clock project. Around. The. Clock. It's not that they are hard to fulfill, but you are fulfilling them without the opportunity to do any of them yourself, and that's where it gets tricky. If I had a list of things for parents to remember to do, it would be for you to also Eat, Sleep, Pee, Poop and occasionally Shower. I don't care if you burp. Presumably you can handle your own gases.

PREGNANCY BY GEOGRAPHY

BECAUSE MATH IS FUN

Question: If a pregnant woman spends 99% of her time in doctor's waiting rooms, but it only feels that way until labor starts when she spends 307% of her time in the triage section of the hospital, waiting to be admitted to give birth after spending 14% of her time shopping for cute clothes online to avoid questions from strangers in addition to 0% of her time in the driveway for First Baby's Car Seat because oops forgot we to install it and an additional 0% of her time in the driveway for Second Baby's Car Seat, because we had a police officer do it once we remembered to buy one, again, plus 74% of her time staring at her own stomach watching Baby TV, also known as "Wow There's an Alien Trying to Bust Out of my Stomach"...

What does all that equal?

Answer: Whatever you like because none of it matters once the kid arrives.

ADVANCED MATERNAL AGE

OR, THAT'S JUST RUDE

I was thirty-six the first time I gave birth. At that age, my mom had three school age children and she started later than everyone else she knew. With my second child, I was an ancient forty-two years old.

I am not suggesting I was actually of an advanced maternal age. But it does get drilled into your head, because sometimes it matters so the docs have to assume it matters all the time and so forth. But hey, if you are one of the young pregnant moms out there – good for you. I guess that means you have a bouncy uterus and your fetus is having more fun than mine. Or maybe your cervix is like, super stretchy! Or maybe your eggs are just a little fresher. Like, mine are the last two left after the last dozen you bought, and yours just got yanked out from under a chicken. Either way, I don't really think it matters – but the medical community is deeply concerned. Deeeeeeply concerned. And that's fine – anything that gets a doctor to truly pay attention to you is a gift. In a pregnancy context. In any other context it's a nightmare. You never, ever want to be the interesting case. Trust me. I won't pretend my medical issues aren't a little odd. I have a sun allergy that causes a skin reaction that makes me resemble a lobster, but only for forty-five minutes until my skin cools. Turns out I am not in fact a zombie, but I may be a vampire. Apologies to the readers of that other book of mine. And this one, come to think of it.

I know people that planned their pregnancies, worked out how old they wanted to be when the kids graduated, all that. My life is a little less coordinated, on top of which I spent my twenties and thirties starting companies and traveling. Which is why I now spend the better part of my afternoon in the pickup line at school. Or running to the store for a birthday present for the kids whose party we missed because the invite was at the bottom of the backpack under a layer of Cheezit dust and snot rags. Everything about my life right now tells me I'm supposed to be old. Even the mail I get. The catalogs feature women wandering serenely on beaches in flowing yards of fabric, presumably looking for a place to use the fabric as a shelter for the Red Cross or a check station of the New York Marathon. Wander, smile. Wander, oh look a shell. Don't bend down you might snap. Wander. We elderly provide a backdrop for all the young moms actually having fun at the beach. Message received – cover your body and walk near the waves. Or perhaps they sell fabric. I don't know. I took one look at Flo McFlowy Clothes and chucked her in the bin. Ageism aside, the idea of having a child in my twenties was laughable. I'm not entirely certain I knew how to tie my own shoes, never mind teach someone else how to do it. Point of fact, I didn't want to tie anyone's shoes, and still don't. Flip flops are far superior for wave wandering.

Advanced Maternal Age means you get to enjoy lots of extra tests and genetic counseling, the main purpose of which is to terrify you into never having sex again lest it result in a pregnancy at an Advanced Maternal Age. All of these delights were afforded me at the age of thirty-six, and like a good little first-time mom I played along. But I wised up for number two at age forty-two and didn't bother to go. Instead, my little girl and I shopped the catalogs for some flowy clothes and built a fort out of them under the dining room table. Thanks, ageism, those floral housecoats have really come in handy!

AN HONEST BIRTH PLAN

Dear Universe:

I would like to have a healthy baby with as little pain to myself as possible, in a setting with the best medical care available which I will have no need of, followed by a quick recovery, no stretch marks and something caffeinated, preferably gallon size, as I gaze at my child who will be the first in history to actually do everything within the "normal" time range.

And if it's not too much to ask, I'd like this to happen no later than the due date but not before it's safe for the baby and only if the crib is already built and we remembered to put the car seat in the car.

Thank you,

Mama Bear

SEE WHAT HAPPENED THERE? Over-reached. Everybody gets stretch marks.

THE PLAN: THE ORIGINAL PLAN, THE NEW PLAN, THE REVISED PLAN AND FINALLY...

THE REVISED NEW PLAN

My plan, for the birth of my second child, was to have my mom out to our house. She would hang with our five-year-old while we were off with the arriving alien. Human. That was The Plan. The Reality occurred three weeks before my due date. Oh, I didn't go into labor, but my mom (quite rudely and with no regard for The Plan) came up with some medical issues of her own. Even went so far as to need surgery, couldn't put it off. Some people have no respect for The Plan. I should mention, we live a mere plane ride away from our nearest relatives. Which was not part of The Original Plan, because our cross-country move came forty-eight hours after we learned we were pregnant and twenty-four hours after we adopted a new puppy because I wanted to be done with potty training a dog well before the arrival. So. The Original Plan was amended to The New Plan, which included packing a house for our cross country move while Lovely Hubby was in a city for the entire summer on the opposite coast. Not the one we were moving to mind you, so we had to look for a place to live online and over the phone sight unseen. I finally arrived in our new city five months pregnant, spun in a circle and picked an obstetrician. It was much like the game Spin the Bottle had I been cool enough to play it as a child. I was cool enough to play it in a gay bar in San Francisco but that is an entirely different book. That's not true. I did play Spin the Bottle in a gay bar in San Francisco, but I actually wasn't cool enough. Where was I? Right. Plans. The Original Plan also had my mom coming out to visit and care for the kindergartener whichever coast we were on. Not happening. We need a new plan.

No problem, right, ask a good friend, a good neighbor? Yes. Excellent idea. Unless you recall that we were new in town by a few months, moved cross country to get there, didn't know a soul, and asking, "Hey do you think you can watch my kid while I go give birth to another kid and we won't be able to give you any warning as to when that will happen" just isn't something I was comfortable with. Honestly, I'd have suspected anyone who agreed to such ridiculousness.

On to The Revised New Plan: Ask Lovely Hubby's mom to fly out. Perfect! That will be great. Yes, she can come. Yes, her flight arrives at 9:30 a.m. on the 11th and the baby isn't due until the 14th. So much time! At 5 a.m. on the 11th, with the baby still safely ensconced in my body, I decided to tempt fate.

"Oh, this baby is so accommodating, your mom gets in at 9:30 this morning, lucky us no early arrival for this little one."

Exactly eighteen minutes later I had the first contraction.

Note to self: "Keep all such smug remarks to yourself."

Self: "Got it."

Lovely Hubby zipped off to pick up Grandma, we threw her out of the car to watch our daughter, continued on to the hospital and all was well with the world. But I can't pretend I planned that! None of that is on me, none of that is good planning. That's just dumb luck. To say otherwise would be to deny how very little we are in control.

Things were a bit more casual when I arrived. My mom was at the doctor on her anniversary with some contractions, but he felt an anniversary wasn't a fun day to have a baby, so he suggested she go home. A few days later, she walked up to his office. We had cars back then, I'm not ancient, she just preferred to walk. As it was not her anniversary, he agreed it was a reasonable day to have a child. Told her he'd meet her at the hospital, which he eventually did but only after I was born. As for my mom, she walked home, did some gardening, washed the dishes. Somewhere in there she recalled a baby was on the way and somewhere in here I'm thinking maybe I should take this personally. She called my dad and once he got home, they headed for the hospital. La di da, off for a summer drive.

"Honey?"

"Yes?"

"Do you think we should have a name picked out?"

"We did pick a name. Kirk."

"Well, what if the baby's a girl?"

"Hmm."

Drive drive drive. No rushing for my dad. This is a man who considers "completely ready to go" sitting in a chair with his shoes and socks near his feet, his shirt unbuttoned and his wallet waiting for him upstairs on the dresser. As he snores.

"The baby could be a girl."

"Kimberly."

"Just as a backup. He's definitely a boy."

I still don't like to be predictable.

While we're here, a quick word on names. I strongly recommend you consider the way my parents did it. Not at the last minute, but alone in a car without input from other people. It takes most of us longer than a casual drive to figure out a name for our offspring. And I am definitely not suggesting that you do what they did, which is have three children whose names all start with K. I'll wait while you work that out.

Got there? Yeah. Email me if you didn't. It may say something about the improved state of our world if you don't know what I'm referring to. I feel very strongly about keeping the name of your child to yourself until introductions are made in person. That way, you can simply say, "This is Joe" and it's a done deal, there is no choice but to love it. If you are on the other side of the conversation I'll reiterate, there is no choice but to love it. That is your role at that point, to support the sleep deprived parents in one of many decisions they have to make. No eye rolls, no harrumphs, just play along. Do not ask "Why did you name him Joseph John Bradley Jake Bellissimo Geranium Fabric Softener McGillicuddy Daniels?" even if "That seems kinda long." The only real response to learning a new moniker is either "I love that name" or "Great name." Great can mean many things, it can mean great and you love it, or great in the huge and terrifying way that a war is "great". Either way, it's still great. If there's a story with the name, the parents will tell you. Asking for it, is just… asking for it. It takes many couples a long, long, long time to come up with a suitable name. Just love it. They can't do anything about it now, and it is what it is until the little human decides to tattoo something else across their forehead.

GENDER

Defined: noun The female or male division of a species, especially as differentiated by social and cultural roles.

TRUE STORY – I PUT "FEMALE" first in that definition. The dictionary, for some inexplicable reason, put "male" first. The dictionary should know better, so I changed it to alphabetical. As it should be.

ALSO, who's asking and why do you want to know?

OH, HUMANS WITH YOUR SILLY GENDER ROLES. YOU ALL TASTE THE SAME TO US

SINCERELY, THE ALIENS

My parents used to joke that they had three kids, one of each. I'm still not sure what that meant. It could have been a reference to my being a 'tomboy' which in those days was a way of distinguishing girls who acted girly and girls who acted human. Oops. Sorry, see that? Totally judgmental there. Frills still don't excite me, but that doesn't mean they can't excite you – oh lord this is exhausting. All opinions are my own. Don't be so fragile. Dang it I did it again! Anyway – I got them back. I used to announce that they were married on the 20th and had their third child on the 22nd – much to the delight of whoever was at the dinner party that night. Not a clue what I was implying of course, but that didn't stop me from being precocious. Dinner parties, by the way, were what family in the burbs did in the seventies in wintertime. In the summer it was barbeques but you can't do that with three feet of snow on the ground.

Gender comes up immediately after due date on the list of required questions, right before the questions about where the fetus has applied to college and if it knows any publishers. That last might just be me. Everyone will be deeply concerned over whether you are having a boy or a girl. Probably because it's one of the more polite questions to ask when someone is pregnant, as opposed to, say, "When was the last time you pooped?" It can be a bit much though. Here's an actual transcript of a conversation I had multiple times while pregnant, usually with strangers:

"Are you having a boy or a girl?"

"We don't know."

"Why not?"

"We like surprises."

"But how are you going to prepare?"

"We plan to love, feed, and clothe our child regardless of gender."

"But what color _____ will you get?"

"Whatever is on sale."

"But, no, really, what are you hoping for?"

"A puppy."

Turns out having a puppy is more difficult than it looks, particularly if you're human. The single most brilliant means of out maneuvering the early gender roles is to dress your infant in Halloween costumes on a daily basis. I can't take credit; it was one of those things that run around the internet gaining likes and laughs. But it is a genius solution.

"Is your baby a boy or a girl?"

"Clearly my baby is a pony in a stormtrooper hat with lizard feet and a rainbow firetruck briefcase. Why do you ask?"

Why do we ask? What is the huge concern over gender? It's really an archaic throwback to when men could own property and women couldn't. It's as simple as that. You own a penis? Congratulations join the landowners over here in Happyville, no, no, doesn't matter if it's large or small you are all winners. Every single time you have to check a box for your child (and there will be thousands of opportunities) consider asking why? If it's the doctor asking, sure, penis owners will have some different medical things going on than vagina owners. And I suppose it matters if you want to think about how you pee, but the truth is men can pee sitting down and women can pee standing up. Not saying it'd be pretty but given the lack of aiming skill in evidence in my bathroom, I'm betting most women could do just as well.

BOYS WILL BE BOYS

A SHORT PLAY

Cast: A Boy and The World.

LIGHTS UP

"Boys will be boys."

"Huh?"

"It means you will only ever be a boy."

"Well, I was hoping for a little more than that."

"Sorry. You are your penis. You are therefore predetermined to have four traits, all of them annoying in general."

"Wish me luck?"

"Luck won't help. You're a boy. You're screwed. Of course, there's always the chance that you will take this in another direction, an entirely patriarchal 'I don't have to be responsible for my actions because after all, I have a penis and you know, boys will be boys' type of thing.' As if you are entirely incapable of making decisions and therefore incapable of being responsible."

"I can make decisions."

"Sorry. Your penis is in charge."

"Makes me sound dumb. And kind of like an asshole."

"Correct."

"Oh. Well, I guess…I guess I'll go shoot some aliens."

"It's not like you have a choice, son."

Lights fade to black.

Thank you for attending this performance of *Boys Will Be Boys*, sponsored by the Committee to Make Sure Everyone will be Forever Limited by their Genitalia.

WE INTERRUPT THIS BOOK TO BRING YOU...

TEN QUESTIONS I NEVER THOUGHT TO ASK, BUT TURNED OUT TO BE REALLY IMPORTANT

1. Will you listen during my ultrasound when I say I don't want to know the gender?
2. How many days each month do you actually deliver babies?
3. Do you consider episiotomies a requirement of birth?
4. Will the birth of my baby have to be worked into your schedule?
5. Would you consider your attitude toward Caesarian Section to be... a) casual b) enthusiastic c) reverent or d) all of the above?
6. How soon after birth will I be considered qualified to hold my own baby?
7. When you say the hospital has a breast-feeding specialist, does the specialist actually support breast-feeding?
8. Will your staff jokingly refer to the pain of circumcision, or are they not total fucking morons?
9. When do I get to eat after I give birth?
10. No, seriously, who is going to make sure there's a tray for me after I run this marathon? And how much caffeine will there be on it?

CAUTIONARY TALES

PART I

I adore medical technicians. Truly I do. I've had the bad fortune to be hospitalized and the good fortune to meet dozens of really caring individuals, who made me feel like an individual. And then there was the ultrasound tech for my second child. Granted, I was grouchy, because a two-hour wait in a windowless waiting room will do that to you. She insisted I couldn't possibly know what I was looking at with my mere mortal eyes. Early on, sure, ultrasounds can be fuzzy and may or may not be footage of aliens on the moon. But this was a few weeks shy of delivery. This was plain as the face on the screen, which happened to be adorable if a little squashed. I'm not a genius; it's just not that difficult to identify the four chambers of the heart when they are pumping away in front of you clear as day. Yet she insisted that I did not know, could not possibly know what we were looking at. Let me clarify, if my baby had a label, I could have read the brand name. In utero sponsoring. It's going to happen.

"You can't possibly know what you're looking at."

"You know, penises look the same in black and white, right?"

Apparently not. Apparently I'd be utterly flummoxed by the appearance of an appendage between the legs of my child. What is that? Am I giving birth to a unicorn? How many legs does this kid own? What is happening?? Oh my word honey we're having an alien!!!

Of the many feelings you can have in a doctor's office, I consider mistrust worse than pain. I really wanted to have a nice look at my kid in utero, as it would probably be the last time. I saw my baby's face, and then I had to turn from the screen, because she refused to tell me where she was going next. It was quite the rude little power play, to be frank. Should I have spoken up? Yes. Did I? Nope. After two hours in a waiting room, I just wanted to get the hell out the door. I left the doctor who sent me to her shortly thereafter. Because if you only deliver babies two days a month, that's really something you should mention a bit earlier in the pregnancy. That and why there's a pickle in my uterus.

(MORE) CAUTIONARY TALES

Once upon a time there was a doctor whose time was more important than mine. She was called many things by her patients and the nurses who worked for her, none of them printable here. We'll call her Dr. Bleeeeep. To be fair, there are a few things working against doctors and they tend to make patients really grumpy. For starters, there's something passive aggressive about being asked to dress poorly and then wait in a cold room for a doctor. Unfortunately for me, I had the last appointment of the day with Dr. Bleeeeep and you know how you get to the end of your workday and just say, screw it; I'll get to this tomorrow? That's essentially what happened to me. Except that I'm a person, and not say, an email or a report. But hey, doctors are people too and they get tired and forget they have patients sometimes right?

No. Not right.

It was my first visit to her office and as she's an OB/GYN, I wasn't terribly excited about being there (even the best GYN visit is still not what we call fun. Entertaining on occasion, but never fun). If you don't know, an OB deals with pregnant and wanting to be pregnant patients and a GYN deals with female reproductive parts, your basic vagina, labia, ovaries, uterine type stuff, whether or not the factory is open. Back to Dr. Bleeeeep.

I entered the frigid room, took off all my armor and put on the ubiquitous paper gown. And then I proceeded to wait for several days. I'd forgotten my phone, didn't own a watch and wasn't going to stick my bare ass out into the hall to see where she was. So I sat there. Freezing.

Since I'm waiting, let's talk about the gown, this garment of invincibility, this last refuge of my naked body, this pretend privacy. It used to be an actual gown, modeled after the gowns used in hospitals. Until it wasn't. It shrank and became a paper vest, and an additional paper napkin was provided to privatize the lower private areas. I can only assume a paper necktie is next on the horizon and the spring collections will feature a couple of shoelaces and a postage stamp. And then weirdly, fabric gowns returned at some places (possible someone understood that throwing out thousands of paper gowns a year might be wasteful? I don't know). In all reality, it should just be a cape – superhero of your choice. I'm going to bring my own to my next mammogram. Because nothing says we take good health seriously like a shiny Captain America™ cape as your boobs are getting crushed. Where was I? Oh, right, three seasons of untold fashion bliss later, I'm still waiting for Dr. Poophead. Sorry, I meant Dr. Bleeeeep. Stuck my head out the door. End of an empty hallway. Not gonna holler. I got dressed, did my hair, brushed my teeth and then stuck my head out, walked a ways and asked a passing nurse.

"Uh, excuse me, where is the doctor?"

I was given the Look, and the Look said, "Holy crap, we forgot you were in there."

I popped back into the room and started undressing again when I overheard them talking in the hall – they couldn't find my doctor. Literally, couldn't find her, so they hunted her down. Based on the conversation, it seems she left and they caught her in the parking garage. Which is fine – absurd, but fine, everyone makes mistakes, oh, ha ha ha, how funny. I can laugh at myself. Clearly. Unfortunately, I also overheard the nurse talking her into coming back to the office to see me. Talking her into it.

"The patient is waiting; you have to come back. Doctor, she's here she's waiting, you must see her. She arrived on time for her appointment and we checked her in and..."

What the? Why is this even a question? At this point, I'd like to say that I waited for her to finally walk in and then told her to go fuck herself, but I didn't. I was due for my annual exam and I'm a good little patient. The fact that she didn't speak to me when she entered, that she literally gave my shoulder a little push to get me to lie down, that she put my foot in the stirrups without saying hello, that she examined me in total silence... I was seething. I was younger. I was foolish. I wanted to get it over with, just get it over with. I'd like to say I asked her what the hell happened to your tongue? Did you lose it along with your watch? But she was about to put a speculum in my body and crank it open, so I opted not to piss her off. The nurse, bless her, was watching me very closely and trying her best to correct the horrifyingly silent examination going on. The current me is still outraged on the younger me's behalf. I later learned that this wasn't simply Dr. Bleeeeep having a bad day. A friend of mine actually had this sorry excuse of a physician deliver her child. And there sat Dr. NoBusinessBeingADoctor, between her patient's legs, mid contraction, about to push out a child, and doc's phone rang. Can you guess? Say it with me now... She answered it. Answered a phone call, while a woman is about to bring a new life into the world, and she is responsible for its health and wealth being.

"Hello? Oh, yes, I'm supposed to be helping someone give birth but I'm way too important to trifle with something as ridiculous as someone's arrival on the planet. Definitely! I am definitely in the wrong profession, no question about that. I don't know how I've managed to keep my license either. But they keep paying me so I'll keep showing up late. All right, oh hang on, I need to catch this kid..."

No, that wasn't what she said, I totally made that up. That's because my friend couldn't tell me about the phone conversation, what with the giving birth going on. As for myself, sometime after our first appointment her nurse called and told me I'd need a follow up based on the tests, and a biopsy that couldn't wait. I simply refused to see her:

"Under no circumstances will Dr. Bleeeeep ever touch my body again in any capacity. You'll have to find me someone else please. Does she have a partner?"

"I understand completely."

Later, when I was pregnant, one of her partners turned out to be a great OB so I stayed with her office. As I neared my due date, I insisted that they give me a schedule of the doctors on call for the practice. I would have stapled my vagina shut rather than have that nitwit anywhere near my child. Lovely Hubby suggested we go to a different hospital if need be. I suppose that would have worked too.

BIRTH

Defined: *verb,* noun The act or instance of being born. The act of bearing someone during their act of being born. Lineage, or the act of tracing everyone who has been born.

GIVING BIRTH

Defined: *verb* the act or instance of getting a human from inside your body to outside your body. There is some effort required, and you should probably let go of any plans you had for that day or the next eighteen years. *See also* superhero

LABOR AND DELIVERY

And delivery? AND delivery. Oh.

I spent a lot of time thinking about labor with my first child. How would it start? What would it feel like? Would it be gradual, or would it crush me into a ball at the get-go? A teacher at the time, one of my main concerns was my water breaking. I did not want my water to break while teaching. Actually, this was my only concern, a casual attitude born of ignorance rather than courage. Not a clue what lay ahead. In the morning, however, I taught ninth graders. I pictured my water breaking and these poor children suddenly finding themselves in a real live biology video. In the afternoon I taught upper classmen, they'd taken my class for years. They knew me well, so while it would be embarrassing, I could always flunk them if they laughed so I wasn't terribly concerned. They, however, were deeply worried. Unbeknownst to me, they devised contingency plans "just in case" the baby chose to arrive during class. It was sweet and by sweet, I mean terrifying to consider that the newly minted driver in the hand me down Volvo who couldn't park and thought speed limits were suggestions was going to get me to the hospital. I was not reassured by the casual, "No problem, miss, I got this" when I asked if he knew where the hospital was. I can only imagine the music my delicate baby genius would have had to endure en route.

Given the option, I preferred labor and delivery the way my aunt did it – a little back pain and forty-five minutes later, a baby! Yes, this is real. No, it doesn't matter how much pregnancy yoga you do, there is no way to organize your body into doing this. Remember – you are not in charge.

My husband and I attended a birthing class, which would have been great if he wasn't distracted by work and I wasn't distracted by the what that's now? Oh, our plan? Our plan. Here is a copy of our plan, in its entirety:

1. We plan to have a baby.

And that was pretty much it. Oh, we also assume it will take place in a hospital of some sort? And my doctor and husband will be present. And you know. A lot of happiness?

I was in labor overnight before we went to the hospital. We took some long walks around the block, me pausing for contractions, Lovely Hubby certain we had to leave right then and there, which meant immediately going back home so he could spend the better part of an hour picking out music. It was fine, though, I don't like to DJ on a good day and I felt like I might be busy. I popped into the hospital hoping to keep on walking and was immediately strapped into a bed, several tubes and beeping things, and a bag of what turned out to be whoop ass going into my vein. It's true – that "can of whoop ass" everyone refers to? It's actually a bag, and it's filled with the shit they use to induce labor. What's most fun about having your labor 'helped' along is when they don't actually tell you they're administering the whoop ass. I honestly thought it was a saline bag. See, I have a tendency to dehydrate. I'm quite good at it, nearly killed myself by accident. Twice. It never occurred to me that I was getting drugs until they hit my system. Couple that with being a first-time mom and all, I really should have made it obvious that I didn't know what I was doing. Here was the extent of my participation in relieving the pain of my labor:

"Do I really have to be in the bed? I feel much better when I walk around, I can handle the pain then."

"No, that's not true. No one walks around. Please get in the bed you're going to want to lie down."

"OK thanks."

No one walks around? Well, sure thing jellybean, strap me to the bed and let it rip. I was an idiot. Thankfully, I was an idiot thirteen years ago and things have progressed. But if for some reason they haven't, know this – if your body is telling you at this point in Labor that you'd feel better walking, there's a really, really, really good chance that you would feel better walking. Unfortunately, I labored in a unit that was about to get very crowded (eight babies born within a forty five minute span) so individualized attention was left to me, Lovely Hubby, and the Doula we didn't think to hire. Lovely Hubby's brain was about to explode what with the impending alien arrival. I felt somewhat calmer about meeting our baby, as we'd gotten along so well so far, but I was concerned about the epidural. No need to panic you here. That delight has its own chapter.

For baby number two, you'll be thrilled to know that I did a lot a more planning. Unfortunately, I didn't actually decide if I was going for a drug free delivery until we got to the hospital. Figured I'd see how it goes. Here's how it went: I arrived at 11:45p.m. dilated at only 2cm and the child was born at 1:41 a.m. How did it go? Rapidly. Really fucking fast. And given that the baby was fine, and I was fine it went great, but I certainly was not mentally prepared for it. What a ding dong. The moral of the chapter for you is this: prepared or not, plan or no plan, the baby is going to do what the baby is going to do. Do as much planning and prep as makes you feel good and healthy and happy. You can plan for eight hours a day for the entire pregnancy, and things can go sideways. You can plan for eight minutes, say yes, let's go for it, natural birth, and things can be fine. I'm not suggesting either of these. I'm not suggesting anything. The only one putting anything in the suggestion box at this point is your baby. And they don't really suggest. They demand.

What I do suggest is to keep your ears open, because it is super fun is to listen to people brag about how awesome they are going to be at childbirth – and how perfectly their husbands are prepared to coach. So cute. I was in the OB waiting room with a couple on their due date. My husband and I were due the following day, and I had some stuff going on. Stuff as in very early labor, soreness, etc. We had a bag packed. I think. Maybe. Could have been groceries I forgot to put away. Our friends in the waiting room though? Wow. This couple was in the World Cup of childbirth. They were on it – stop watches and lists and bags and plans to be best buddies with everyone on the ward so someday their child could literally have lifelong friends. That's a really charming idea when you think about it. A little hard logistically, but very heart felt). And the birth itself? Her husband/coach was ready, steady, gonna make it all a breeze. Had we spoken longer I can only assume we'd have the invite for the baby's eventual wedding, bride side please. Why, yes, they knew the parts their baby would have, I mean come on! Planning!

I hope that's how it went. I truly do. I was right there cheering them, go, go, go right up to the point where she was concerned because it was four p.m. and the birth announcements they'd printed had today's date and she thought maybe she'd have to have them reprinted. Um. Yeah. The baby is in charge of the schedule. That's just how it is. Unless you are having a C-section of course, and then you have the unenviable task of picking your child's birthdate. Me? I'd have the C-section in say January but pick a summer birth date. Then walk around with my six-month-old and freak everyone out. Red shirt that birth!

COME ON IN THE WATER'S FINE

When I was born, the doctors used what my mom calls "twilight gas." It sounded strange even before the word twilight was welded to images of vampires and werewolves. Her description was thus, "they put a mask over my face, I was unconscious, then conscious, then you were coming, then I was unconscious and I swear the doctor wasn't there then I woke up and the nurse handed you to me." I was born at the very end of the sixties, so who the hell knows what was going on. Sounds a bit trippy, but of course, I did my bit as a new alien, wailed on cue and haven't stopped babbling since.

Babbles are one of the happier sounds of pregnancy and birth. Like the gasps when you find out for sure, the oohs and aahs when the baby does something cute or heroic, like burping. The delighted sighs that accompany labor pains. Wait, what? For my first child I made absolutely no preparations for actual delivery, so sound didn't really come into consideration, though we did have some great music playing. For my second child I was determined to have a real plan, or at least an idea. Or like, put some thought into it ahead of time. Probably. Anyway, I knew I wanted to have a different experience if I could. I thought I might like something a little more au natural.

I know, all childbirth is natural and I'm fully supporting of natural childbirth. I'm fully supportive of any type of birth where the baby is healthy and the momma is happy. Honestly. I don't care where you are if it all works out. But I've noticed, and perhaps you have too, that there are those rare occasions when humans have just the tiniest tendency to out-do ourselves? Outpace our own well-being, as it were? At any moment, I expect the extreme births to begin. Kids born in orbit so they can continue to experience the weightlessness of the womb as they round the far side of the moon. And of course if your child isn't floating in space when they enter existence you may as well have L-O-S-E-R tattooed on their forehead because they will Never Ever Be All That. Before we get there though, let's talk about water births. I had a new gynecologist after a move, and she asked about the births of my children. When I told her my second was a water birth, she said, and I quote:

"Oh. You're one of those moms."

Never having been one of "those" anything, I was simultaneously proud and confused. Here's how it all went down:

- At twenty weeks pregnant we moved cross country
- At twenty-one weeks I grabbed the first OB I could find, because I needed someone, being of Advanced Maternal Age and all
- At thirty-four weeks I discovered that she only delivered babies twice a month. I'm not sure you're an obstetrician if you deliver only twice a month. You definitely aren't a pizza service.
- At thirty-four weeks and a day I found a midwife, who happened to specialize in water births.

And that's why Lovely Hubby and I found ourselves in a water birth class when our second was well on the way. Let's go around the room and introduce ourselves.

"I'm about 25 weeks."

"I'm about 22 weeks."

"I'm due next summer."

"And Kimberly?"

"I'm due on Thursday."

This was on Sunday.

Yup. Really planned this one out. It's not entirely my fault what with the last minute doctor change. There I was, a few days away from popping. Ravenous, of course, pretty much the entire time. And I had to have my feet up, because—right swelling. OK, my feet weren't actually swelling but my mid-wife was making very sharp remarks, so I had to act like they were.

"Oh, your feet should be up, you know, if you feel you need to. If anyone is in need of putting their feet up, go right ahead. If there's not enough chairs I'm sure your partner will be happy to hold your feet. Don't be shy. Get those doggies up."

Stare stare stare.

I finally put them up just so we could back to the videos. We watched several films of water birth. It was magical. I mean this sincerely. Everyone in it had long hair, the women, the men, the children, the camera operators, everyone.

The scene opened on a shot of a large tub with a clear side. In it, a woman floating, mermaid-like, hair in drifts on the surface. The back wall was made of stone, probably hewn from a quarry run by tiny elves, or perhaps the warehouse staff of IKEA. Very natural, very pine needles in my hair and the scent of fresh water. Scene after idyllic scene of women with mermaid hair floating, floating. Occasionally one of these beatific birthing moments would include a man in the tub with the mermaid, presumably the baby's father. They didn't specify but it would be a little weird if it were someone else, just one woman's opinion. The merman, who also enjoyed flowing hair and a flowing beard, calmly discussed in the voice over how he can feel the pain of her contractions radiating through the water and he'd take on some of that pain into himself. Share it with her.

Uh huh.

And there were several of these really remarkable, peaceful, almost trancelike videos of women, just gently floating in the calm water, their mouths a perfect 'o' as they quietly breathed in and delivered their little mer-people, all the while leaning, ever so slightly, against their partners. One couple who showed up multiple times, so I hope the births were a few years apart, for her sake. Unless her merman took on all that pain for her, then you know go for it. The second and third videos of them included their little children, gently splashing in the water, the whole family naked, as she again, ever so gently gave birth. And I thought, as I'm sure you did, I hope it's warm in there, those kids are going to get cold.

Finally, because floating in a Plexiglas pool surrounded by a fake rock wall isn't actually nature—yes. You guessed it, well done. The last birth video was outside, merpeople in a pool of water sweetly kissed by a brook while birds sang and the inhabitants of Narnia gathered in reverence... Fine there were no talking beasts. But they were outside in a brook/pool type thing. Which is kind of fantastic in a very, very, VERY retro Garden of Eden way. Of course, Eve didn't give birth in the Garden of Eden because you know, Catholic guilt.

It was lovely. We sat in that room, lulled into a trance by the birth-giving mermaids. Eyes glazed, our thoughts pooling into peaceful little waterfalls. Sigh. And I do adore water, swimming during my pregnancies felt wonderful. Very comfortable in water. On top of which, my mid-wife worked out of a hospital. The water birthing suite was inside a regular maternity ward, so should anything go wrong, Lovely Hubby wouldn't have climb out of a swimming hole and hike down a mountain to get help. Seemed great. And it was, it absolutely was great. So great. So very great.

The thing is, and I didn't realize it until much, much, much later, like a year after my son was born—the sound was off. The sound was off in the freaking videos. We were listening to quiet little tinkle tinkle music and lullaby voiceovers done later in some studio of course. These women appeared so stoic, so gently, quietly heroic. Maybe they were. It's possible. But maybe they were screaming their freakin' heads off. Because I was not quiet. I. Was. Not. Quiet. And I'm OK with that- the baby already knew I was loud, he'd been listening to me for nine months.

It started in the hall outside the water birthing suite. After nineteen hours of contractions, I got to the hospital at 2 cm and an hour and twenty minutes later I had a baby in my arms. If you're reading this before you have a baby, don't worry- yours won't be that fast. That's crazy painful. If you're reading this after you've had a baby – yes, your labor was much worse, I had it easy. There I was, standing in the hall, waiting to go into the delivery room. Standing by choice, I'm sure they would have let me sit down but I was afraid if I bent my knees I'd be giving birth in the hallway. Why did I have to wait? They had to fill the tub. They can't fill the tub until they know you're going to be the one using it, which they determine by like all these little tests when you get there. So I'm in the hallway chanting ever so quietly:

"Fill it fill fill it fill it fill it fill it fill it fill the fucking tub just fill the fucking tub the tub the tub the tub fill it fill fill it fill it fill it fill it fill it fill it fill fill it fill it fill it fill it fill it fill the fucking tub just fill the fucking tub the tub the tub the tub fill it fill fill it fill it fill it fill it fill it!"

Remember the mermaid women? So calm, and quiet, and just the slightest little wrinkle to their smooth foreheads... their mouths a perfect "O" during transition labor for just a moment, then back to serenely smiling? I was exactly like that. Delicate really, and so calm. I remember my mid-wife saying, "Uh, Kimberly? Could you try to be a little gentler with yourself? You know, like yoga." I was attempting to knock down a wall with my head to distract myself. Honestly, next time, I'm just going to have the kid in space. Keep it simple.

LABOR PAIN

Defined: *noun* Must be experienced to be understood. Sorry penises.

Euphemisms for Labor Pain which aren't fooling anyone:

1. Pressure
2. Surge
3. Butterfly Kisses
4. Nuclear Bomb
5. The Shredding
6. Sweet Mother of God My Body is Being Torn in Half

E.E.E.K!

Enemas, Epidurals, and Episiotomies. Eeek!

Ah, yes, the trifecta of delightful procedures that you may or may not participate in when you give birth. You may be concerned, or even be afraid of these things during childbirth. Or you may not have thought about them at all and if so, I apologize for bringing them up.

Let's start with the one that concerns me most – the episiotomy. You thought I was going to say enema, didn't you? I did too, but turns out, the episiotomy has me freaked. As with all things related to birth – there are a few ways of looking at it. The baby is going to exit through a hole which, despite its best efforts, is likely to fall short of the mark. And since we're all giving birth to geniuses with presumably big brains, well, you see the problem. So, what is an episiotomy exactly? It's a cut. You know that tiny bit of real estate between your vagina and your butt hole? Well, it's going to just about disappear. Not entirely. But pretty close. Oh – if your doctor is a frequent slicer, be sure to ask what degree is used most often. There are degrees to these slices – so you could be, you know, nicked just a touch or you could be opened wide. And this is a procedure that for some doctors and hospitals is an absolute standard 100% every single time no exceptions. At least, at one of the hospitals I toured.

Lovely Hubby and I were having our second child and having moved cross country again, we did the local hospital tour. We wandered the halls with maybe five or six pairs of first-time parents. At question and answer time, I asked how soon after birth I would have my child in my arms. I was told "well, you're going to be recovering from your episiotomy and getting you know, fixed up (i.e., stitched) so you're going to want a few minutes." Which begged the follow up question, "Why would I be getting an episiotomy?" "Oh, everyone does." Everyone? "Yes. It's part of the procedure." I could only assume that the 'procedure' we were discussing was the birth of my child (cue angelic singing). I looked at the other parents to be. Everyone was nodding, everyone was smiling, everyone was happy. Everyone gets a slice, like pizza in the break room. Yippee?

I did not get an episiotomy with either child. Both times my child was helped out by the combined efforts of me and the doc/mid-wife with no slices. As described by Lovely Hubby, my doc had her arm in me up to the elbow. So truly, I know not whereof I speak, but I do know that not everyone has to get an episiotomy.

Epidurals are another option, for an entirely different reason. The pain of childbirth can be absurd. There's really no other way I can describe it. I have no equivalent, though I've seen video of experiments in which the abdominal muscles of men were put through a similar spasm, induced by a machine sending signals to their nerves. I think one of them lasted like seven minutes and the other forty-five. This isn't because men are wimps. It's because that shit hurts like nothing else. Not for everyone, of course, and certainly there are people who breeze through it. My aunt's labor for all three kids consisted of a little back pain and forty-five minutes later, there was her baby. Now, if we could order what type of labor we get, I'm sure everyone would go something a little less painful. But no matter, it is what it is. Oh, and there are people who will tell you that you can overcome your pain and this and that and the other, and maybe you can. Maybe you can't, but maybe you can. It's really not for anyone else to say. With my first child, an epidural was perfect for me. I was in the hospital, as I mention elsewhere, hooked up to labor inducing drugs, to 'help me along.' As no one told me they were giving me Pitocin and I was too giddy to even ask what was going on, I was enjoying a chemical induced, hyper increased version of labor. Kind of like sitting in a chair one minute, and the next that chair is falling down an elevator shaft, while someone punches you in the face. Like a poorly written action movie.

I wanted to walk around to ease my pain, but I was told, oh no, no one walks around during labor. No one! Yes, this particular nurse was perhaps in the wrong line of work, or at least the wrong department. I went along with it – what did I know? Everybody said listen to the nurses, they've seen it all a million times. That's true. And most of the time that's probably great advice.

I'm told that the pain of induced labor does not have the slow build, rise and crest of a natural labor pain. Having experienced both, I can say that it didn't make a shit bit of difference to me- induced or not, the pain sucked incomprehensibly.

My doctor arrived, asked if we were living in the dark ages, and inquired of the nurses why I hadn't been offered an epidural? I believe I said yes before she finished her sentence. Now, let me tell you, I was afraid of the epidural, not because it's a needle (it is) and not because it's huge (it is) but because I was concerned that I would have a contraction in the middle of it and twitch or move or something and then there would be a problem with my spine (it's injected into your spinal cord or near your spinal or close enough for mere mortals to call it your spinal cord). First, I never saw the needle. Good. Second, I was told to sit up and swing my legs over the side of the bed, I think I was leaning on a nurse, and Lovely Hubby was behind me presumably making sure everything went OK. I'm not sure, my eyes were closed, and I was breathing as slowly as I could. Breathing in for a slow count, and out for a slow count. And it was over. That fast. And the relief was immediate and absolutely fantastic. I believe I promptly dug my tiara out of my bag of essentials and took a nap shortly thereafter. We're going to have to wait on that enema.

WHAT TOOK SO LONG? ARE YOU STILL IN LABOR?

Well, we would have been done hours ago, but I ate a cheeseburger and it's sitting in my lower colon, and the kid just can't get his head around it. Which brings us to our third "E" ticket ride – the enema. Now, I have to be honest, the idea of having a tube stuck up my butt, filled with water, and flushed out did not appeal to me in any way. Why would I want something additional stuck into my body when the whole point of giving birth was to get things OUT? Why would I want several gallons of water added to the bloat I was already carrying? Why would we be messing around with my butthole when my birth canal is just around the corner and has a child coming out of it? Real estate, that's why.

In her infinite wisdom, Mother Nature put the exit for the birth canal right next door to the exit for the digestive system, which means that internally, your uterus sits on top of your colon. Hmmm... Now, don't get me wrong, I adore Mother Nature. The engineering on the human body is mind boggling (see my other books). The engineering on growing a baby, well, that deserves at least its own section (see elsewhere in this book.) But the colon has the potential to be quite...full. And the birth canal, presumably, is going to also be quite full around the time you're giving birth. So. You have a colon full of delicious pizza remnants. Delicious when they were eaten, I'm not suggesting they're delicious once they're in your colon, though I'm sure there's a dog somewhere that would think so, and probably someone on the internet somewhere has ideas about their tastiness. Certainly there are microbes and other organisms that would describe colon contents as divine given the option and the ability to speak. Anyway – your colon is full of poop and your birth canal is full of baby. Since the baby is going to come out anyway, perhaps it's best to make room for it.

For baby number two, I agreed to an enema. It was so much worse than I thought it would be. But only during. Afterwards, I can say that it definitely made a difference. Let me walk you through this. When we finally got into the water birthing suite, it was time to loosen things up wink wink. They peeled me off the ceiling and had me on all fours on a hospital bed. Because we were working with a midwife, Lovely Hubby got the honors of holding what I can only assume was a 90-gallon tank of water. It was behind me, so I really have no idea. Or perhaps they were emptying the tub they just filled into my ass. Tough to say. So there I am, with no idea what to expect, because I didn't bother to research what an enema actually is, I just knew tube into butt, add water and that was going to clear out my colon, thereby making more room for my pelvis to open, thereby making more room for the baby. You're basically rearranging the items in the fridge and gaining space by finally tossing those containers of what used to be food. So, there I am on all fours, stunning hospital gown hiked up around my hips. I have a moment of relief from the pain as the shift in position puts the baby hanging below me instead of being carried by my spine. Tube goes in, and warm water bathes me. I'm thrilled because any sensation that isn't pain is welcome. Then my midwife pipes up:

"No, you have to clench your butt."

"What's that now?"

"You have to clench your butt. You have to hold all the water inside."

What the fuck? I have to hold 90 gallons of water inside me ALONG with the baby? Couldn't I just let it all go and maybe the baby will come out in the wash, so to speak? No? Clench up? Oh dear god.

Let me put this in perspective for you. Imagine you need to have the largest bowel movement of your life, and force feeds you a Vegas size buffet, so you've got it from both ends. Now, you're bare assed, so your body thinks, hey, it's poop time, but it's not. You have to hold it. And you have to clench your butt closed as tight as you can. Just for fun, let's see how long you can clench your butt for. Start now, I'll see you in a few chapters…

Oh, but it gets worse. So much worse.

She sends Lovely Hubby off to the car to get the rest of our stuff. I learned later she tells them to leave the suitcase behind for the specific purpose of getting the partners out of the room at this particular time. So he's gone. She then tells me, go into the bathroom, but don't go to the bathroom. Great. I have to clench, not push my baby out because it's not time yet and walk across the room to the bathroom. Right.

Do you know how hard it is to change positions while your butt is clenched? Try it. I dare you. Get on all fours up on a table, because you're on a hospital gurney when they give you the enema. Now clench your butt as hard as you can—a little harder—keep it clenched as you climb off to a standing position. Don't let go! Squeeze. CLENCH HARDER! Now without giving birth or letting go of your rectum in any way, slowly ever so slowly walk across the floor to the bathroom. With me so far? Let's make it a little more realistic. Please repeat all of that but do it while you're having contractions. DO IT! Sorry. Little transition labor anger there.

Me, my enormous belly, and my clenched butt climbed gingerly off the bed, shuffled across the floor, did NOT look at the toilet for fear that would signal the brain to signal the rectum to let loose, and carefully turned around to stand in front of the toilet.

Here's the lucky part – the bathroom was just the toilet, a tiny little closet with close walls, so while I was standing there specifically not pooping, at least I could put a hand on each wall to hold me up. Which was hugely lucky, because of what came next. Ready? Still clenched?

"March."

"What the fu-raaaggh frigging freak what the my god ow."*

*It should be noted that like children, contractions have no concerns about interrupting your conversations.

"Don't push Kimberly. March."

"I'm not… I don't… did…did you say… march?"

"Yes."

That's right, because there's nothing else going on, you have to march in place. Churn up all that water. March in place, knees high, clench my rectum tight, oh, and it's not like labor just stops for all of this fun, I've still got massively rolling contractions, oh excuse me 'surges' or even more foolish, 'pressure' beating the piss out of me, and all I really want to do is collapse but I'm marching and clenching and marching and holding on and clench and don't push and ow ow o wow and march and pain and clench and get those knees up and squeeze and there's a band practice about the break out for crying out loud—She pops her head into view to ask how I'm doing.

"Oh, you know. Not a lot going on. Perhaps I can do your taxes while I'm in here?"

"Super, keep squeezing."

"AaaaghAAaaAAAghAAACccAAAAGh!"

Finally, finally, she tells me I can sit down, and you know what happens the moment I bend my knees. This is why the partners are asked to step out and get the suitcase at this moment. Because no one needs to see ninety gallons of water explode out their beloved's butt, along with the remains of every meal they've ever eaten. Remember when you were a kid and people said if you swallowed gum it stayed in you for seven years? That's true. Don't ask me how I know, but it's true.

The tsunami continued for quite some time, with intermittent bouts of marching in place and butt clenching, and all this happens while I'm going through transition labor! Poopapocalypse 2012 did subside before Lovely Hubby returned. I don't know how she got the timing right, but that midwife really knew what she was doing. Just get me in the tub. Get me in the tub! Please!!!

She cleaned me up, and presumably the entire bathroom was nice and sparkly, and he was none the wiser. Not that it would have mattered. Lovely Hubby is nothing if not practical, and the human body doesn't faze him in the slightest, no matter how pedestrian the activity. And finally, finally I was able to get into the tub. We had just a few moments til baby time.

"You're going to feel a little pressure" is the second greatest understatement I've ever heard from a medical professional. The other also involved my vagina but it's in that other book, the one with the stuff that hasn't happened yet. Prequels are weird.

My little merman was born, kicking his legs in the water and having a grand old time. Snuggled up under my chin, and that was that. Oh, there was that moment when his shoulders got stuck and we considered giving him a scuba diving course given how long he'd been underwater, but I tend to gloss over the scary bits all these years later when the bambino is happily healthy.

SLEEP

Defined: *verb* Experience whenever possible *i.e., Her every waking thought was concerned with sleep. She was too tired to see the irony.*

THE SCHEDULE

Babies must be kept to a schedule from the moment they are conceived or they become unruly tyrants who want to do things like eat and sleep whenever they want. That's absurd, we can't have children deciding what they want, how could they possibly know what they want when a commercial or product placement hasn't told them yet? Which reminds me, please make sure your kids see as many commercials as possible. An entire generation of seventies children were traumatized because due to lack of commercials. Everyone was watching PBS.

Your baby just arrived on the planet, so as a parent your job is to be their personal assistant while simultaneously trying to get your alien to conform to your pre-ordained schedule. Also, there's a worldwide panic that the new parent will somehow forget the alien needs food and sleep and fresh dipes. Mainly because no one else wants to be responsible for the diaper part. The scheduling concept is therefore drilled into the heads of new parents on a regular, well, schedule. Like so:

VARIATION ONE:

Me: "I'm pregnant."

The General Public: "When is the baby due? We have timetables that must be adhered to and I'd like to offer you some advice based on what I know about a person sitting inside the uterus of someone I've just met. Let me tell you what you should be doing."

VARIATION TWO:

Me: "I'm pregnant."

Friends & Family: "Great! When are you due? We're going on a cruise next summer."

"Great! You know, it's important, it's important, keep the baby on a schedule or they'll never sleep through the night."

"It is, yeah, that's important."

"Has anyone mentioned getting the baby on a schedule? It's important."

"Do you have a planner?"

"Important."

"So critical."

"Really need a schedule. Don't blow this off. I'm looking at you, Kimberly."

"We use a BabyBit for ours!"

"Ooh! The BabyBit! Is that one with the..."

"It's the important one. For the scheduling."

"Yes, it tracks sleep, measures the amount of food ingested and also comes with a scale so you can weigh diapers to check the amount of pee wee pee pees and poopie doos coming out."

Me: "Never mind."

I swear to you, my child will never have pee wee pee pees or poopie doos. I don't care how important digestion is. The focus of The Schedule will be sleep. That's not because food and diapers aren't important. It's because as a rule, the General Public won't offer to breast feed your kid and as a rule, your Friends & Family will diaper if need be but don't want you thinking it's a regular thing. Now, I'm not suggesting that sleep isn't important, it is. I'm useless without at least 14 hours and an afternoon nap. However. How many adults do you know who sleep through the night? Be honest. How many people do you know who lay their head down to rest, fall asleep instantly, and pop back awake a luxurious eight hours later? At this very moment it's 2:40 a.m., I'm wide awake, and my kids haven't been babies for years.

You should think about having your child on a sleep schedule; it will give you something to focus on other than the total lack of sleep you're getting. But here's the thing (oh please, Kimberly, tell us the thing. I will, thank you very much). The thing is – it's going to change. Whatever carefully calibrated schedule you create for your little human is going to change after, at best, two weeks. At worst, forty-five minutes. In which case you may not have gotten the little jerk on a schedule and maybe you just managed to get them to sleep for a bit. Either way, nothing is permanent. There are no permanent solutions. My sister describes it thus: With a child, you are constantly helping them to form habits, and then break those habits. Also, you can't teach them everything all at once. Probably because they are way smarter than we are and are likely laughing inside, "Oh, look at the adult human trying to so hard to make me do this or that. Why would I bother? She will do it for me. Good human."

All I'm saying is, before you blame baby for the lack of sleep, consider what you were getting before. Presumably you were involved in some kind of sexual activity, possibly taking place at night. Not necessarily, of course, but possibly. I'm told that humans do have sex during the day. I would not know, being long married and occasionally confused when Lovely Hubby sleeps in the bed. Assuming of course he can successfully remove whatever child/pet giraffe/pile of laundry has wandered in.

THE FOURTH TRIMESTER

Ever wake up with your head resting gently against the wall in your hallway, still on your feet? No? Just me? Oh you thought the hard part was done when the baby was born? So did I! The fourth trimester has two major things in it – first your baby, and thank goodness for that because the second thing is a lack of sleep so profound it seems impossible. I kept waiting to pass out. If you go weeks on end, with no more than two consecutive hours of sleep, at some point you wonder – why haven't I collapsed? What is this physical impossibility? And then you wake up, standing in your own hallway. Could have been worse. Could have been the grocery store, closing your eyes for just a minute with your head in the cart until you slam into something and it wakes you up in time to drive home...

Sorry. Dozed off.

I did in fact wake up one afternoon leaning against the wall in my hallway. Not possible? Wrong! It happened. I walked from my bedroom to the nursery down the hall. There was something urgent I needed to get to in there, but I can't recall what it was. I opened my eyes to find myself at a slight tilt, shoulder resting gently on the wall in my hallway. Huh. This is potentially embarrassing. I seem to be asleep standing up.

The level of exhaustion associated with a newborn child is limitless. Perhaps you will be fortunate, and your baby will sleep for hours on end with little or no issues. You must never tell anyone. Ever. Ever at all. No one will like you. Everyone will consider you either a liar, a braggart, or both and that your child is either drunk all the time or the Spawn of Satan, angelically waiting for the right moment to take over the world. No, no no. Don't do it. Don't tell people. Shh. I don't care how much you want to brag. Just don't. I once worked in a tiny office which had an exceptionally high percentage of employees pregnant at the same time (yes, many jokes about what was in the water, insert your own here _________). The first to give birth was a real go-getter, well liked and quite popular. Unfortunately, she made the fatal errors of 1) an easy birth 2) telling people about the easy birth and 3) the audacity to show up at the office when the tot was a week old with fresh baked cookies. This was all well and good until the other first-time moms started to go through their own labor and delivery. Lulled into a false sense of security by the first woman's easy peasy lemon squeasy new mom life, the reality was that much more difficult to bear. Outraged and sleep deprived, the other women in the office revolted. The first mom was ostracized, required to bring cookies every week just to get anyone to talk to her. I was single and childless and perfectly content to eat the cookies, but I remembered the lesson: Keep the cookies for yourself, because the people at the office are awful.

Likewise, never ask the parent of a newborn if the child is sleeping. You will know if the child is sleeping, because if the little darling is, then the person you are talking to is also asleep to take advantage of that five minute window, and all you are doing is disturbing their much needed rest with your pestering, foolish question. Furthermore and in complete contradiction, do not instruct the parent to sleep when their child sleeps. This is absurd. Unlike some moms (hint hint, office mom I mentioned in the last paragraph) most new parents are just trying to get through one box of diapers at a time, and correctly gage when the new box needs to be purchased. This is enough for a sleep-deprived mind. I once attempted to sleep while my daughter slept. She was snuggled in for a nap, and I thought, why not? Why not try it and see? She was in a Moses basket, right next to me for fear of 1) me rolling on her and 2) she could in fact be the Second Coming, so it seemed appropriate. Ego notwithstanding, I thought, I'll do it. I'll lie down, and I'll sleep whiles she sleeps. I'm doing it, I'm going to try… try… it... sleeeeeeeeep…sleep…

Deep, peaceful rest cocooned me in deliciousness. I rolled over, stretched, sleepy smile, huge yawn.

"Man."

Yawn.

"What a nap."

Refreshed, recharged. I felt dreamy and energized; I bounced off the bed and glanced at the clock. Three minutes. I got three minutes of sleep. How desperately deprived do you have to be for three minutes of sleep to give you a spa vacation result?

Sleeping children, of course, are angels. Why so precious? Because this is what you have at the end of the day. This is how you manage not to kill your children while they are awake, because at night, asleep, they seem so peaceful, so gentle, so absolutely perfect. You drift off to bed, blissfully steeped in enough love to get you through the vomit and the nightmares to come. Later, later. Right now, breathe deep and tuck them in. This works for any age, by the way. I totally caught my mom watching me nap. May have been because I was supposed to be picking up the kids from school at the time, but I still looked cute. In all honesty, it seems a bit creepy to me now to think of my mom watching me sleep as a kid. But I don't think that happened in the seventies. Our parents weren't as concerned about us breathing. They figured if we survived the day, sleeping should be a snap.

PLEASE SLEEP CHANT

FOR YOUNG BABIES

Kind of like a haiku, but with more angst:

Sleep sleep sleep sleep
Please oh please just sleep
Sleep sleep sleep sleep sleep.
Sleeeeeep Shhhhhh Sleeeeeep
That's right... shh... sleep little
Oh frig! He's awake...
Shh... Shhhhhh...
Sleep sleep sleep sleep.

Repeat until the child outgrows whatever is happening.

And then suddenly, this happens:

One night Lovely Hubby and were getting our daughter ready for bed. She was just around eighteen months and our only child so it was still a project. We put her pj's on her, something adorable with feet I'm sure. She looked up at us and said, "Bed." Lovely Hubby and I thought, uh, OK. So we put her in her crib. She looked at us and said, "Book."

So we gave her a book. She looked at us and said, "Bye." So we left the room and cried for a half an hour. "Bed. Book. Bye." That was it.

THE NIGHT NIGHT MEDITATION

FOR TODDLERS AND OLDER CHILDREN

At some point your child will graduate to a "big kid" bed. There's a reason cribs have bars. Sleep chants (see previous sections) will no longer suffice. You're going to have to call on all available powers.

Begin approximately 6 ½ minutes after you've put your child to bed for the fourth time. So after a glass of water, after a bathroom visit because of the water, and after those other two random pop ups out of bed. Repeat until you pass out asleep on the floor of your child's room.

> Deep breath… and…
> *Wait, why are you out of bed?*
> *No, why are you out of bed?*
> *Didn't I just tuck you in?*
> *You just had water.*
> *You just had it.*
> *Fine.*
> *Here's your water.*
> *Now go to sleep.*

Take three deep breaths... and...

Hold, on, why are you out of bed?
Didn't I just bring you water?
What's wrong with your covers?
That's because you keep jumping out of bed.
Jump back in.
NO! Not literally, you'll hit your head on the top bunk.
OK. Are you in bed?
OK.
Goodnight.

One deep breath and
What? What are you doing out of –
Of course the covers are messed up.
You keep jumping-
I can't remake it while you're in it.
Come out of bed.
I know I told you to stay in bed,
But you asked me to remake it and I can't do that
While you're in it.
Yes. Nurses can do that.
I am not a nurse.
It would be useful to learn, yes.
I don't know how to become a nurse,
At school I guess.
All right?
Good night.
I love you too.
Sweet dreams to you too.
You are tucked in.
No you can't have a book you're sleeping.
Goodnight.
Goodnight.
Goodnight.

Deep breath–nope-
Oh sweet mother of god why are you out of bed?
No, never mind, it doesn't matter.
Just go to bed.
Just go to bed.
Just go to bed.
Goodnight.
Sleep tight.

Deep br- grrrrr
What the hell?
Get in bed.
Bed. Bed. B.E.D.
Now.
Now.
Now.
There is no tomorrow if you don't get in bed.
I am going to stop tomorrow.
Yes, I'm that powerful.

Deep breath as child reappears.

Point at the bed.

Continue to point at the bed as you breathe deeply.
Deeper.

Namaste.

PLAN

Defined: *verb* To arrange a scheme for. Honestly, there's no point in even trying to be clever here. Your days of planning are over. Everyone who asks you about your kids' schedule is in on the joke. Don't be fooled. Sorry about that other section. Didn't mean to mislead you.

A WORD ON CONTRACEPTION

YES

"Apologies for the wait – the doctor is in the middle of a delivery and will be right back." The over packed waiting room relaxed, no point in getting upset. We'd all just had babies or were about to, so waiting was old hat. As I had my own baby in my arms, I could afford to be magnanimous with my time. After all, I was there for my six-week sex checkup. Yes, the magical moment six-weeks after birth when the doc hopefully clears you to have sex again. The nurse popped her head out twice more before I was able to get in -- apparently the delivery was taking so long because the mom was having triplets! Little known fact, the word triplets! is required to be followed by an exclamation point, in print and speech. Time passed quite quickly then, as I thanked every god I could think of. I know I was not nor ever will be the person to try and manage multiples. I can barely manage to remember to feed myself. I was still rolling that image around in my head when it was my turn with the doc.

"I heard about the triplets! – is everyone OK?"

"Everyone is fine."

"I hope the mom has some support, a lot of family around?"

"Unfortunately, she's alone. Well, not alone. She has a nine month old baby."

I was rendered speechless at that point, likely as shocking to you as the doctor's announcement was to me. She continued with the exam, of course, all in a day's work for her.

"So, Kimberly, everything looks good, it's ok to be active again. What would you like to do for birth control? Kimberly? Birth control? What would you like?"

"I. I'd like…all of it. All of it. Give me everything you've got."

Remarkably, the modern-day chastity belt is quite comfortable.

DIVIDE AND CONQUER

You will be approached, immediately upon having your first child, with questions about your second. That's correct. Before your uterus has even resumed its original shape, someone is thinking about putting it to work again so enjoy that ten or twelve minutes right after your kid arrives. At some moment in the very near future, the idea of a sibling will come up. If it doesn't happen prior, your child will bring it up the moment they realize that there are such things as little sisters or little brothers and that they could be bigger than someone. I've heard that siblings are sometimes planned or even scheduled. Not in our house mind you. We moved to California so we wouldn't have to keep track of what season comes next. But I do feel siblings are worth thinking about. In fact I am going to ask you to carefully consider the number of children you have, not because of overpopulation or some environmental concern, simply this:

Do you want to be outnumbered?

That's it. With one kid, you can double team the little alien. Otherwise, you run one on one defense with equal numbers of parents and kids in the family OR you run a zone defense. Lovely Hubby and I opted for one on one defense, but I know lots of families with a gang of children and they always seem to be having a good time. Personally I can't find my washing machine behind the mountain of laundry so I'm not sure how that part works out for them.

Perhaps you have one child and you're thinking of having another? Maybe primo was great and you want to see if you can hit the jackpot again. Maybe the first child really sucked, so you want another go. Maybe you'd like a shot at the other gender. Maybe you've done this five times already, but you love it and want to raise more children. Maybe you're trying for a matched set. Maybe you're like me and you think your own siblings are the best. Maybe you have deep concerns about over population. Maybe you can only have one child. Maybe you'd like to but can't have children. Maybe maybe maybe maybe it's nobody's damn business, except your partners', why you have the number of children you do. Including zero. If you opt not to have zero, the general public will try to convince you to have another to keep your alien company.

Ah, siblings. Siblings are an undeniable blessing and a curse. There's probably a reason the first family discussed in the Bible included sibling rivalry on a violent scale. No one is closer. Closer to your DNA, closer to your experience of the world, closer to being able to understand where you come from because "hey, them too!" There are many members of my family who do not have siblings (my dad for one) and it's definitely changed things for them. I have a beautiful relationship with my brother and sister, aided by the fact that we rarely live in the same time zone. Perhaps if we lived closer we'd squabble more. It seems a double-edged sword. Live close, fight over dumb stuff. Live apart, can't share the fun stuff. My youngest refers to any day spent with his cousins as Cousins Day. As if the whole nation is also celebrating his almost next of kin. We're heading to a reunion this summer. His head may explode.

When it came to siblings, Lovely Hubby and I employ the one on one defense because we weren't foolish or brave enough to be outnumbered by our children. I heartily salute anyone who is. God speed. Sibling relationships are so complex, they deserve another book. Written by someone else. Because my children love each other, but also regularly reject each other wholeheartedly and with great cruelty. They can arrive at the breakfast table mere seconds after waking and already be in a full scale argument. About... daylight? Breakfast? The hallway? No idea. They also spend hours devising elaborate games that can be played by two children with a six year age gap.

So, really damned if I know.

What I do know, from my own childhood, is that divide and conquer is not simply a useful parenting strategy. Divide and conquer is also an excellent way of dealing with parents, so beware. I was an expert in rerouting parental attention away from me and onto each other. A word here, a mention of this or that, and boom, they were off in an argument of their own and I was off entirely the hook. I believe the pundits call it deflecting. Which reminds me, when two or more children are in a family they immediately form a law firm whose sole purpose is to maintain detailed ledgers of slights, pardons, favors and treats as distributed among the siblings with intent to justify additional treats or favors for each individual partner in the firm, while maintaining a general accounting of mistakes, gaffs, and faux pas committed by the "parents" and any breaches of the ice cream contract, as described elsewhere in this document. All promises are binding, and the legal terms contained herewith have no relevance whatsoever except those created under the Tree House Conventions of 2015, commonly known as the "It's Not Fair" referendum.

See? Don't let them get together. Divide and conquer.

IN LOVING MEMORY OF ANYTHING (ANYTHING AT ALL) THAT HAPPENED IN THE MIDDLE OF THE AFTERNOON

Oh thing that happened
In the middle of the afternoon
While I was working
Or perhaps relaxing
But definitely awake
I miss you.

I miss you deeply
Or perhaps not you, thing,
So much as the timing of you
So perfect
So thoughtful
So accommodating
The middle of the afternoon
While I was at a meeting
Or running an errand.
But definitely
Assuredly
Awake

Unlike everything
That has ever happened
Since I became a parent

Oh thing, how I miss the kindness of your timing
Awakened now
In the middle of the night
Or when I've just drifted off to sleep
By a medical crisis
Or a really good idea for a Halloween costume but three years from now Mom because you know I already have the next two planned
Or vomit
Or it's cousin, the poop that never ends.

I never appreciated you, thing in the middle of the afternoon.
Bleary eyed, caffeine deficient.
I never knew how good we had it.

I wish I could have you back.
Relive those carefree days
Of dealing with crises
During daylight.

Farewell my friend.
Farewell.

SMOOTH

LIKE CHUNKY PEANUT BUTTER

As your kids get older, there's a myth that the planning becomes easier. Oh dear. By this point you've been lied to so many times, it probably feels real. I know it did for me. Which is why, as the parent of school age children, my favorite, favorite, F-A-V-O-R-I-T-E advice is when I'm told to plan ahead, to make ahead, to have everything ready by the door. Uh huh. Good idea. Here's how that works in our house:

Everything is set up the night before, lunches packed, backpacks near the door, clothes neatly laid out for the next morning.

AND A NEW DAY DAWNS...

The six year old is ready three hours ahead of time, and proceeds to unpack his backpack all over the house, eat the snacks from his lunch and simultaneously put on and lose his sweatshirt.

The twelve year old picks put the best outfit ever, only to find in the morning that her hair isn't doing what she wants, which changes her hair style, which changes her clothes, inevitably needing to rifle through the laundry for that one shirt she likes to wear when her hair is down, which she can't find and so subsequently yells at the cat, who is being using her favorite shirt as a scratching post/something to suckle and said shirt is covered in cat spit.

At which point the dogs sneak into the room where we keep the cat stuff, eat the cat food (one of them is highly allergic to cat food) as well as the offerings left in the kitty litter while the children scream at each other, because miraculously they are both ready to brush their teeth at the exact same time (difficult to do over a small pedestal sink without someone getting spit foam in their hair) which in turn pushes my buttons and I start to holler because the clock is ticking and we are running late, leading to high stress for the six year old who completely shuts down because he can't find the back pack he took apart when he wanted to read his library book one last time and the we all turn around to see the dog vomit all over the missing backpack while the cat runs for the litter box trailing what can only be last night's leftover spaghetti from an undisclosed orifice.

Good thing we had that all set up the night before. Parenting books, like tidying books and financial advice, work about ten percent of the time if you're lucky.

Even so, if there's a baby there's a biological imperative to plan, nest, make cozy, hyggee - which is a Swedish word meaning "look at what ridiculous Americans will do to pretend they have a lifestyle, we took some candles and a sweater and created a movement. How jolly."

It's possible I'm paraphrasing.

PARENT

Defined: *noun* A father or a mother, a progenitor, or creator, a source, origin or cause. *The parent of sibling rivalry is, of course, the parents of the siblings.*

see also COMPETITION *noun* The acting of competing, rivalry. Oh, you have no idea. No idea what you are in for. I'm laughing too hard to be helpful. Or am I? Maybe I am. Or maybe I'm trying to gain an edge for my children by not giving you my best advice.

ONLY NINE CIRCLES OF HELL, DANTE? STEP IT UP.

Welcome to the show. Oh, not Major League Baseball, or even Broadway. Welcome to THE SHOW. That's right. Like it or not, you've entered the arena, where assuming you can survive what is happening in your own house, the entire world is now available, ready, willing and able to judgy mcjudge your parenting skills, style, Insta gallery of pics, and professional play date readiness. So many opinions, so so many.

More than enough, really.

In keeping with Dante's Nine Circles of Hell but obviously making it better, I offer you Basso's Ten Rings of Judgment. There is no "but I'm a good person" alternative here. You can be the greatest parent in the world. You probably are. Doesn't matter. Someone, somewhere is judging you.

Basso's Ten Rings of Judgement

First Ring: Your Parents

You are doing things differently. Clearly that means you think they did it wrong but truly the way they did it was better. Sorry.

Second Ring: The Family

Either because they are raising their kids according to family practices or they aren't, either way, you are doing it wrong. Also, you never returned that dish.

Third Ring: The Friends

They are raising aliens as well, but they are raising aliens according to their family practices. Or against their family practices. Doesn't matter. Their way is better.

Fourth Circle: The Neighbors

Granted, they watch you stand on your front stoop because your toddler locked you out of your house when you stepped outside for the mail. Again. You'll never do it right.

Fifth Circle: The Strangers at the Beach

They watch you chase your buck-naked child for ten minutes as she laughs her head off because she stripped down when she got caught in a wave. But at least they're laughing. Much preferred to *The Strangers at the Grocery Store* who are in such a hurry to get their shopping done but not so much of a hurry that they can't lecture you with their eye rolls.

Sixth Circle: The Strangers Online

Raising their children according to a religion, a political stance, or a meme. All three have about as much to do with your child as, oh, I don't know, the avocado sitting in my fruit basket. What do you mean you don't keep avocados in the fruit basket???

Seventh Circle

Who the hell really cares at this point?
Honestly, is no one else having a difficult time?

Eight Circle
Fuck it.

Ninth Circle: Your Own Child's Siblings
You're supposed to raise siblings in a manner identical to each of the siblings prior regardless of how much time has passed and anything you've learned, so you're trapped forever in a system that doesn't account for experience, knowledge, or change.

Tenth Circle: Subset to all but the First Circle
People who don't have children but know exactly how yours should be raised. Don't worry. Dante has a circle for them too.

Not only will you be judged, you are required to compete. Please select from the two types of competitors, those who compete via one-upmanship in a superiority way (my kid is smarter, faster, bigger, smaller) and those who don't care which direction the scale is headed, they will compete: "Suzy is having some trouble with spelling" is met with "We're quite certain Johnny will be in jail before he's two and indicted on racketeering charges by seven, he's that much of a delinquent."

In addition, you are now busier than you have ever been. It doesn't particularly matter if you are actually busier. You may have a whole village of people helping you or maybe your kids are low key. Regardless, you are busy. But whatever you do, don't actually say you are busy because—

"Wait what, did you just say you're busy?"

"Busy? Who's busy?"

"That's nothing, I worked overtime this week and went to three baseball practices!"

"That's nothing, I started a company, visited orphans overseas and did it while recovering from back surgery."

"I see your back surgery and raise you a mother-in-law with gout, a turtle stuck in our chimney, an international incident between the space station and my teen who wants to be a hacker, and a fight in the school parking lot."

To be topped only by Marjorie. Dearest Marjorie, who is so busy she fell asleep while using the cross walk to usher not only her children, her neighbor's children, and several exchange students into school, but managed to stop an incoming mini-van with her prone body, saving all those kids in her sleep and sustaining major injuries as a result. Marjorie wins. Marjorie, whose Last Will & Testament included detailed instructions on how to run the school bake sale and a forty page dissertation on what kind of peanut butter is best for baking, versus sandwich making. Thank you for your contribution, Marjorie, rest in peace.

I wish you the absolute best with all of that. Having spent the better part of my youth with a competitive spirit that can only be labeled self-destructive, I've chosen a different path as a parent. I know, I know, I'm supposed to be deeply concerned with what other people think/have/want. Been there, done that. Oh Kimberly, you think, how could you be competitive to the point of being self-destructive? As a child? That seems difficult. Actually, it was quite easy, and as you'll see, my excessive competitive attitude was something I needed to curb, for my own sanity and health.

Allow me to elaborate. I once ran through a six-foot-high wooden fence with my face. Oh, you're thinking, that's not competitive, that's just weird. Fine, I'll elaborate some more. The fence was made of one by eight inch board, placed flat side between posts. It was also the finish line of a race. I leaned in to win, full speed and smashed the board with my face. Split the board in two, ended up with the top half of my body hanging over the boards below that didn't break. Did that with my face. So I could win. It happened at a birthday party meaning there was literally nothing at stake. In the seventies they did not reward every moment of every child's life with an ovation and the keys to a new car. And thank goodness they didn't – because the bragging rights alone were enough for me to tear open my cheek with my glorious face smashing victory. Hell yes I won! That my friends, is a competitive spirit. Did they call an ambulance? No. Did they call my parents? No. This was the seventies for cripes sake, they stuck a pack of frozen peas on my rapidly swelling face and moved on to cake time, because it was cake time. Nothing stops cake time!

Given my predilection for competitiveness and my ignored potential as a martial artist (uh, anyone can break a board with their fist, losers, try doing it with your face) the adult me carefully removed all instances of competition from my life. Which is why I'm a writer, because it's not like they make Best Seller lists or have designed an industry with a thousand gatekeepers and a mere chosen few rise to the top. How absurd. And horrifying. That would be like giving out a Pulitzer for writing.

The pressure to be a competitive parent comes early, it comes hard, and it comes from all directions. Sometimes self-created. But mainly other pregnant women, in a never ending quest to reign superior for puking the most, gaining the most weight, gaining the least weight, (how dangerous is that), ankle swelling and my personal favorite – how much do your boobs hurt and how many times did you actually poop over the course of your pregnancy? Zero? You get second place. There's a chick in New Hampshire who ate nothing but cheese since 1983. Actually, you both lose.

The good news is that just because other parents are competing with you, does not mean you have to compete with them. Truly, the best defense is no offense. I'm not always grown up enough to accomplish it, but if someone is in full brag mode they are either a) genuinely happy about the little tyke or b) genuinely insecure about the little tyke or c) some combination thereof. How to manage it? Say, "That's so cool. Wow. You must be very proud, three full diapers in one day?"

or "Amazing! I'm certain she did recite the alphabet at four and a half weeks" or "I know he's going to be a NASA engineer; I did see him throw that plate on the floor to see if gravity works! I will definitely vote for her/him/them!" On second thought, that might come off as slightly snarky. Just say, "I read that's a sign of increased intelligence, what a smartee!"

Now if this little one is your first child – don't even attempt it. Just avoid other first children. I mean this. I once listened to an ongoing dialogue on the wonders of Timmy as his motor skills drills were described in detail so he could be the first in his family to walk before eight months. To be followed, I assume by a round the world trek, as he walks the earth like Johnny Appleseed spreading his gummy toothed smile of joy. Let me help you with this, everyone out there thinking it's so cool the first time your kid walks. Walking is infinitely more annoying than crawling. Why on earth would I want my child to walk as soon as possible? That just makes her more mobile and harder to keep track of. Is no one else lazy?

I'm fairly certain my parents noticed I was walking at some point. I know Lovely Hubby's realized it when he came home in a police cruiser. He was about two, walked out the front door and was found by a neighbor. The officers picked him up and brought him home. He popped out the back of the cruiser and headed back into the house. Much to the surprise of his parents. See? Walking is dangerous. What if he tripped getting out of the cruiser?

School is an excellent place for nurturing competitors, as long as you don't let education get in the way. When I went to pre-school, it was entirely voluntary, rarely used by anyone except those with working moms, and led to the completely optional kindergarten. That's right, optional kindergarten. Like, don't even bother to show up and eat paste if you don't want to, these construction paper doodads will be fine without you. Not true for me now as a parent. By pre-school age, the competition has gone through several rounds and is heading into its finale. No joke. Because if you haven't Worked It All Out before

Pre-School Your Child is Clearly Done. With what, I've no idea. There are areas of the country that seem, well, we'll say more prone to this kind of thinking. You can also read this as there are areas of the country where people are actually this bat shit bananas.

Shortly after my third cross country move, my little one and I visited a park. Standard, neighborhood park – swings, climbing thing, a few benches, dog poop left behind. As a rule, parents talk to each other. Standing there, deciding which slide to go down, you already have something in common, so you chat. It's also, unfortunately, an excellent opportunity to compete and to judge and yeah.

"Honey walk around the swing, so you don't get smacked in the head. No, around – walk around—around it. That's not around it's right in front – OH. Oops. Ouch. Guess that wasn't far enough. OK does that hurt? A lot? A little is you need an ice pack maybe, and a lot is say, a hospital. A kiss? OK, a kiss. Done. Good job you. Have fun."

"She OK?"

"She is."

"She really shouldn't go down the slide head first. She's going to get hurt again."

"She probably shouldn't – oh and yet she did."

Pause as the shock of that reality sits. I could see it looping through her brain, 'she shouldn't have, but she did, she shouldn't have, but she did.' Luckily she spoke again before something in there broke.

"We haven't seen you before, did you just come to the neighborhood?"

"About two weeks ago, from back East."

"The Valley?"

"No, the East Coast. Miami. How about you, are you from around here?"

"Oh. Yes, I am, grew up here. So how old is she?

"She's two. Well, two and a half. Thirty months? I guess I don't have to say months anymore."

"Where is she going to high school?"

"Oh she's not doing pre-school until maybe next year, if I'm not working at home."

"No – I said High School."

Pause while my brain plays it over and over, 'high school, high school, high school.' Luckily she spoke again before anything in there broke.

"High School. You know you have to decide now, so you can figure out where she should go to middle school, so you know what elementary to go to and that will tell you what pre-school to apply to."

"Ah. OK. Well. Let's see. I haven't found the grocery store yet, so the grad school application reverse engineering process is back burnered."

I told you, I try to be a grown up about this stuff. I didn't say I was successful. Luckily, all she heard was engineer.

"Ooh, I know just the pre-k for engineering."

"Oh, thank you, really, that's OK. We're OK. We're going to take it slow."

I must have ruffled a feather, because here's what came next:

"Honey, is that your Uncle Jay on the billboard? Look honey, it's your Uncle Jay!"

I assume at this point I was supposed to ask who Uncle Jay was but given that his face was twenty feet tall on a billboard about some movie, I went out on a limb and guessed that he was in the film industry. I'm astute like that. I took my slightly swing damaged child and headed out of the park. Nah, we didn't exchange numbers to arrange a play date.

HOW YOU CAN RUIN SPORTS FOR YOUR CHILD

It's never too early to start destroying any joy your child may feel in their athletic endeavors. Hard to believe, but there were no organized sports in the seventies. For females. Sorry, forgot that little tidbit. When I was a child my choices were cheering for the boys who played football and... nothing. I did cheer for a season when I was in eighth grade but found I did not enjoy being an athletic supporter. And why would I? I was an excellent receiver and put in plenty of time as linebacker on the neighborhood line. The lack of leagues didn't stop me from playing football, mind you, it didn't stop any of us. We just played in the open lot between two houses without the benefit of pads or parents. The former being a more painful proposition than the latter. Precious little of our time was spent in the company of adults. "Be home when the streetlights come on" was the general rule from parents. And "what they don't know won't hurt them" was the general rule from the kids. After all, it's hard to play Hide and Seek in the dark if you go home when the streetlights come on. It's also hard to let everyone know the streetlights are on if you use the entire block to play Hide and Seek. It's possible that Timmy is still lost somewhere in Mrs. Foley's rhododendrons.

Were there down sides to being unsupervised? Sure. Did we get slammed to the ground and have the wind knocked out of us? Yes. Did we argue endlessly about the made-up rules? Yes. Did everyone play? Yes – truly. No one could be on the sidelines; we needed every player. Did things get broken? Yes, both human things and thing things. Did we play in the street and scream "Car" whenever a car appeared, echoing it down the line "Car CAR cAr cAR," to be followed ten minutes later when that last kid hollered "CAAAAARRRR!!!"? Yes. We had 'do-overs' and a lot of sweat and dirt and occasionally a fight and definitely some bruises. We all played together, one big hodge-podge of ages, attitudes and abilities. No one got a trophy. No one got a ribbon. No one got anything except five minutes worth of bragging rights, erased immediately.

It's slightly different today. My parents made sure the door was unlocked so we could get out and get in and that was pretty much the end of the involvement. At least for me. I do recall playing catcher for my brother who pitched in Little League. Not on his team, silly, just in our yard, I was a girl, remember? If you are planning to have your child participate in sports, it's best to begin planning when the tyke is still in utero, because you only have five years. It's not a long time and the competition is fierce because most college sports scholarships are awarded to kids in kindergarten. Never mind the fact that if a recruiter is at a Tee Ball game, there's a high likelihood they are there to watch their own kid. Don't allow logic to get in the way of your plans. Better get cracking.

Here are a few tips to help you get those sports accolades that your little one has been dreaming of since you were a child:

1. Don't coach, but be at every practice to criticize the coach, your child, other children and everyone sitting on the other side of the field, including that grandma with her really goofy sun hat. I mean come on; this is serious. This is Tee Ball.
2. Decide in utero what sport Suzy will play based on a carefully calibrated timing system of her kicks, rolls and flips.

3. Force your kid onto any team in any sport you choose, regardless of interest or ability.
4. Ignore coaches who think that kids who try out and don't make the cut shouldn't be allowed to play. Do not allow your child to find something they are actually good at – that's for quitters.
5. Stick with only one sport, start at six months old, play year round, and play in multiple leagues with a minimum of two practices per day. Consider homeschooling.
6. To execute number five properly, the child must master the first sport before trying any other sport – mastery includes at least four offers from Division One schools and an endorsement deal. Don't settle for less, loser.
7. If number six is done properly, your child will enjoy a repetitive use injury by the age of twelve that is not normally seen until the age of forty. It can happen by ten years old if you are any good at parenting. Are you any good? ARE you? ARE YOU? Too slow – GIVE ME TWENTY REPS.

As you can imagine, the coach who works with your child is going to be really important, after all, they are the source of your child's future scholarships, professional team placement, income and what's that other thing? Oh, right, happiness. Sometimes, if you aren't competitive enough, your child will play a sport that you don't have to try out for. Three year olds often fall into this category, because three years olds are notoriously lazy about off-season training. This simply means you aren't serious enough about parenting, and you need to re-prioritize in order to effectively destroy your child's love of sports in a more efficient manner. If you find yourself in that situation, the coach becomes even more critical.

Coaching criteria for maximum destruction of sports enjoyment:

1. ONLY WORK WITH COACHES WHO SPEAK IN ALL CAPS.

2. Only work with coaches who mock the other teams.
3. Only work with coaches who decide in the first three minutes if your child is any good at the sport, and talks to them according: "Well, Sport, you can't throw, or catch, or pitch, or hit, and I know you're only seven and played tee ball once, but it seems like you haven't been training in the off season. When was the last time you were in a batting cage? I'll give your mom a list of equipment she can purchase to help boost you, but you can't really play, so I'm going to put you in the outfield, and then when you do something great, I'll take credit for it, because you were such a loser when you got here."
4. Only work with coaches who foster team spirit by asking the other players, "What did Sport do wrong?"
5. Only work with coaches who can't be bothered to remember anyone's name and calls everyone Tiger. Kidding, those guys are LOSERS. Call everyone Sport.

Got it? All righty! Play ball! Oh wait, beware of Existential Gold Stars. These are things your child will receive in lieu of actual accolades for actual, child specific accomplishments. They often take the form of trophies that you will have to dust.

WORST PARENT IN THE WORLD™ POINT SYSTEM

If youth sports aren't competitive enough for you, i.e., you win every fist fight over bad calls and you've been banned from 78% of the fields in your hometown or alternatively you have no athletic skills whatsoever but still have something to prove, you've come to the right place. Lovely Hubby and I would like to suggest our pride and joy, the Worst Parent in the World™ Point System:

- All events must take place with at least one of your children.
- The appropriate response to any child's eye roll, disgusted snort or overemphasized sigh is an immediate super loud, up high in the sky high-five with your partner and a declaration of the points you've earned. If they aren't with you, call them and discuss the points you earned as loud as you can. Open the windows so the neighbors can share your victory.
- Foot stomps are worth ten points each, so count off by ten as they tromp down the hall. Out loud of course. If you can work them up to a door slam at the end of the stomp double your score.
- Feel free to get creative – children like nothing more than

when their parents fail them in ways they can talk to therapists about later.

Here's a small sample of events so you get a sense of it, but really, it's a free-range system and we invite you to have some fun. I know I do. You may want to start slow, a few items a day until you get the swing of it:

- Leaving an infant behind when you go on vacation (I'm looking at you Mom and Dad) is worth one thousand points, with bonus points if you get back before the baby knows.
- Lying to your child for convenience can be worth anywhere from ten points to hundreds of points, depending on the age of your child. Lying to toddlers is only worth a few points; after all they are so gullible. Bonus points if you can make up some utterly impossible and keep them believing it until they are in their teens, like carrots are good for their eyes (it's total BS, look it up. Also, the Brits are quite good at this game, just saying).
- Asking a child to eat a vegetable, brush their teeth or go to bed at a reasonable hour are all excellent ways to rack up points on a daily basis with little to no effort, and when they are older you can double the points if you also have a daily breakfast they need to attend and/or want them to wear shoes or a coat to school.
- If your decision to **not** to buy that toy/candy/unidentifiable desired object results in a full-blown toddler tantrum with maximum judgment from strangers, congratulations you get as many points as you'd like. Double bonus points if you can induce this kind of rage in a child over the age of seven.

As your children get older it's more difficult to annoy them in some ways (they have ear buds in and can't hear you) and easier in other ways, because you after all, you breathe. Here's a little teen preview, in case you'd like to start planning:

- General embarrassment for a teen is worth some points, if it's done at full volume in public. The eye rolls in your kitchen may be strenuous enough to sprain something but they aren't worth a lot of points, so save it for the special visits to the school cafeteria. Or better yet, the locker room. Of the opposite gender.
- Friend specific teen embarrassment is worth a lot if it involves multiple sets of parents, grandparents and at minimum three types of social media.
- For maximum "special friend" horror, pretty much anything can be done with your underwear on your head. While dancing. To oldies.

There is a leaderboard, but we opted not to include it. It just didn't seem fair, as Lovely Hubby and I are thousands of points ahead what with our fourteen year head start. In fact, we've accumulated 573,228,494,683 points. Today.

I'M BUSY OLYMPICS

The layers of competition don't end with home life and activities, school age children offer a myriad of ways for their parents to compete. My parents were spared much of this, because they, like all the other parents we knew in the seventies, were not involved on campus. They weren't trying to make up for a lack of art, music, or physical education. They weren't holding book drives paper drives and bake sales to raise money for a new roof. It's almost like those things were part of our public schools *anyway*. Today, well today things are just slightly different. We'll focus on one area where parents can compete, I mean support schools: the average school parent group, or Parental Torture Association. There are two kinds:

- The fun kind that run like a soap opera, with villains, heroes, lovers and liars in which absolutely nothing gets done but there is a high level of entertainment value
- The functional kind, which is a group of unicorns and gryphons volunteering at your kid's school.

As I haven't seen any rainbow-colored poop around here (which is a complete lie if you read the whole book) let's talk about the first kind.

Technically, the purpose of a Parental Torture Association is to enable our government to avoid educating an enormously geographic and economically diverse population by relying on bake sales and the fact that parents need their school age children to be educated while they are still school age. No one can wait for the government to fix it, and then our kids age out, and voila, still not fixed. Enter the raisers of funds and providers of all that is creative. I mean this literally, at my son's school, the fundraisers to pay for technology upgrades, the art program, the music program, the dance program, the garden program, the assemblies, the fields trips- basically, anything that you actually remember about elementary school, they're on it. It's equally impressive and depressing. But we're not going to solve all that today, so let's focus on you. How are you going to survive? There are options of course.

1. Ignore them. An excellent choice. Good luck. Not because they're so good at getting you but because I have to ask all you out there ignoring the people who are trying to improve the school your child attends – really? REALLY? Oh, but Kimberly, you promised not to judge us. Fine. Not judging. As long as *you*, and I mean this sincerely, are *not complaining*. NOT. COMPLAINING. No, no no. You do not complain. Step up, or shut up, you cannot have it both ways.
2. Participate. Do one thing. An excellent choice. Good luck. Not because you shouldn't do one thing, you should, if only because it then releases you from the 'no complaining' contract. Draw a hard and fast line around what you are willing to do- then take that line, and line it with dynamite. And a moat. Filled with radioactive alligators and screaming toddlers. And fire. And maybe some snakes or spiders, depending on how outdoorsy your local fundraiser types are.

If you are in group one, good for you. Please write as large a check as possible for you. And remember – no complaining!

If you are in group two, you are in for a treat. What follows the entrance into the Parental Torture Association is a hallowed and sacred ritual known as the "I'm So Busy Olympics." In this multi-year, multi-event, multi-platform competition, busy parents vie for an exciting array of awards, accolades, and medical diagnoses:

- Most Likely to Have a Heart Attack
- Most Likely to forget her own Children's birthdays
- Most Likely to miss a meeting she called
- Most likely to keep a meeting going longer than needed
- Most likely to make the other parents want to kill her
- Most Likely to Be Male (one qualifier yearly)
- Most Likely to Confuse Volunteering with Being Best Friends with the Principal
- Most Likely to Horrify Her Children
- Most Likely to Confuse Her Children into thinking they Run the School
- Most Likely to Alienate Anyone Who Might be Willing to Volunteer
- Most Likely to Pretend She Knows Everything (that's mine and you can't have it!)
- The Last Minute Sprinters Get It Done in Ten Minutes Squad
- Most Likely to Confuse Being a Grown-Up with Being in Junior High, awarded annually to the Clique
- The Assembly / Picture Day / Teacher Appreciation / Spring Carnival Relay Awarded to the same six people who volunteer every event.
- The Worn Out Award – usually given to the above relay team by year 2.

There's really nothing else to say to your local Parental Torture Association, except thank you. And you should probably lead with that.

FEAR

Defined: *noun* A distressing emotion aroused by impending danger or evil. Concern, anxiety. Coming back to the kitchen to find your toddler on top of the refrigerator. Yes, you left him buckled in his highchair. Why, does that matter?

EVERYTHING YOU NEED TO BE AFRAID OF

A BRIEF OVERVIEW

We haven't seen the news today, but this is accurate as of twenty minutes ago:

Child #1: Everything.

Child #2: Life threatening allergies and climate change.*

Child #3: Not so much fear as general unease, "What happens if the kid bumps her head when her concussion is only a week old?" And in my house growing up, "Hey, does anyone know where child #3 is?"

Child #4. No 5. Wait…

"Hey, whose kid is this? Honey, we have someone else's kid in the van again."

"Which van?"

"The van I'm driving. Where are you guys?"

"Damned if I know."

"OK. Stay there."

Don't worry; it's not necessary to actually instill this. It's biological. The moment your child is born, everything is a danger.

*As with all charts, I've included some contradictory information here in small print, just to throw off any interpretation:

It should be noted that I have two children, not including Lovely Hubby on occasion. The information on this chart (child #3+) is based on the downward slide in my parental vigilance from child #1 to child #2. I am regularly reminded of this slide in rules by child #1, as discussed in detail under sibling rivalry in a book written by someone else. My assumptions are probably also rooted in the fact that my own parents forgot me when they went on vacation, and I was their third child. For those with more than two children, I'm sure you are quite skilled and just as vigilant as ever. Well done you.

THE LONG WAY HOME

Parenting can be scary. Books can terrify you (there's a particularly popular pregnancy book that lists every possible disease and what week they get started during pregnancy. I lasted about four days with that one. No thank you). Friends can terrify you, particularly if they have awful children. Your children can scare you, even in utero, there are kicks to the ribs that jolt you awake when the bambino decides to have a dance party at 3 a.m. It is my sincere hope that this book won't terrify you too much, or if it does, it will only be out of understandable concern for my children.

So. You made it through Labor AND Delivery (well done you). Now comes the real test, the real terror. You have to get your child from the hospital to your home. It's time to be released with your young into the wild. What you think you want, when leaving the hospital, is a fully loaded ambulance, a police escort, and armored cars to fore and aft. We got the police escort all right. Wait, let me back up…

When my first child was born, there were eight little aliens welcomed to the world in forty five minutes. That is not an exaggeration, eight humans born on the ward in less than an hour. The nurses were running from room to room. Our nurse even ran away at one point, sorry she couldn't finish delivery (shift change at seven, I'd been pushing for an hour) and ran right back five minutes later. All the better, she was great, and may as well see the thing through. Anyway, so many babies born one after the other after the other. And there are nine million tests that must be done right away. Right away! Every baby is poked, prodded, squished, needled and generally smacked around. The welcoming committee really blows it on the first few minutes of life on this planet, which does not give me hope for when the aliens arrive. My little one was pronounced healthy and the vials of blood taken were promptly left in our room. Instead of say, the lab, where they might have a chance of getting tested. It is completely and totally understandable, eight new humans in forty-five minutes! I can't get eight people to show up for a meeting within an hour of each other. My doctor delivered three of the babies born in that rush. So, yeah, a few hours later, maybe around ten p.m. that night my daguhter's blood got to the lab. No problem, it got there, everything was fine. Lots of juggling of medical results, but all was fine.

Until the day of our departure, when they tell me that I will be going home without her that day.

"All set? OK, your daughter will be staying here but we are ready to check you out."

"Excuse me?

"Ready to go home?"

"Is my daughter going home?

"No."

"Then neither am I."

"Oh. Really? Oh. Well, now, let me see... oh, here it is. It takes 48 hours for the blood work on the heel jab number ninety-five test to come back and it didn't get to the lab until after 10pm the night she was born. "

"That answer is… incorrect. Either I am leaving with my baby, or my baby and I are staying here together."

"Well, she'll be in a very small room."

"Really? The nursery with the 8,000 other babies is a really small room? You know what, no problem, it's completely OK, I don't mind small rooms."

"Well, there's no bed or anything. "

"I'm sure we can scrounge me up a chair. That will be fine for me. I don't need much, but I'm not leaving without my girl."

We checked out of the hospital together at about 11pm that night. Not entirely sure that was protocol, but I didn't care then and I don't now. She was cleared for release so let's get the hell out of here. Which brings me to our drive home, a straight shot of about eight to ten miles down a main drag, then a few blocks over to our neighborhood. When I say main drag, emphasis on the drag. As in racing. Four police cruisers chased a little white piece of crap car up, down, around, over and past us as we went home, me in the backseat huddled over the little one. And when I say raced, I mean he went through the red lights, changed direction, up the other side, cut across lanes, scraped the curb, slammed the brakes, reversed again. It was madness. Sirens, lights, horns, me chanting "Get off this road get off this road get off this road." We were finally able to get away from the car chase, and safely arrived in our little driveway.

"Oh, I know, it's the middle of the night, but we're bringing baby home, Lovely Hubby, can you film it?"

There we were. Me holding my bundle of love, and in the background, screaming sirens and horns. Needless to say the little one and I did not take another trip in the car for quite some time.

By the time she was five years old I was feeling quite comfortable in the car again, even without a police escort. I was pregnant with baby number two and, well I know I promised not to make suggestions—

your baby, your birth. But at this point, allow me to say – don't have a car accident while pregnant. I apologize if that's pushy and I know I'm taking a real risk but avoid it if possible. Not the greatest way to spend a morning. We were driving, presumably, on our way somewhere fun on a Saturday morning. Or maybe IKEA. Me, Lovely Hubby and our daughter. I was twenty-four weeks pregnant, and fully engaged in Baby Brain.

Unfortunately, I was not fully engaged in driving. According to Lovely Hubby, I was fully facing him. Instead of say, the road. As I drove. In stop and go traffic. He must have been saying something really riveting, because I had no response time at all as I slammed us into the back of the SUV just ahead. Well done me. Lovely Hubby got our girl out of the car and checked her while I sat, very quietly, behind the wheel. I felt a little kick in my belly, so far, so good. We decided, after camping on the side of the road to exchange pleasantries and paperwork with my new friends in the SUV, that we should go to the hospital just to have me and our girl checked.

Enter the EMT's. Now, understand, on Long Island, ambulance service is free. That's right, free. Because EMT's are volunteers. As are firefighters. Are you following this? Long Island. New York. Remember all those first responders streaming into the twin towers? Volunteers. I'll give you a minute.

They were quite happy that I'd felt the baby move, but we all agreed it wouldn't be a bad idea to have some additional professionals take a look. You what's not fun? Waiting while the Emergency Room OB tries find your baby's heart beat after a car accident. I waited an entire lifetime in that sixty seconds, covered in cold belly jelly. You know what else is no fun? Realizing after the OB successfully hears your child's heartbeat that the additional three nurses standing on either side of your hospital gurney are not there to celebrate with you (though they do) they are there in case they cannot find the heart beat and you wig the fuck out. There is no fear like fear for your child. Just to be safe, I was told by the head nurse I'd be kept for observation.

Lovely Hubby was found on the pediatrics side of the ER, and cheerily informed that I was fine, but I was being brought up to L&D.

"What's L&D?" asked my non-medical professional husband.

"Labor and delivery," replied Nurse Chirpy.

My husband is a strong man but being told his 24-week pregnant wife was heading to Labor and Delivery was a bit much even for his stoic self. He dropped his color, his phone, and whatever was in his colon as she quickly recognized his panic and her error.

"Oh no, no no – she's not delivering. We're just checking her, going to hook her up to the monitors and make sure she's not having contractions."

Six hours of nothing later and we went home. I didn't drive.

WELL THAT'S TERRIFYING

I'm told the scariest moment for my mother happened when I was six months old, and I didn't make a sound. I fell out of my crib, and all she heard was the thunk. She ran upstairs to find me lying on the floor completely silent. She said it was so much worse than if I'd been screaming. And I did my share of screaming. Like most kids, I was terrified of the hairdresser. You thought I was going to say dentist, right? My uncle was my dentist, so those visits were all bubble gum flavored fluoride and visits with the cousins. No, I was terrified of the hairdresser, because I had no use for a hairbrush. After all, I couldn't see my hair so what did I care what it looked like? But the hairdresser, he cared very much about hairbrushes. And tangles. Every. Single. Yank. Of that brush. Snapped. My head. Back. I wailed. It was painful. It was also an insulting waste of my time. Just shave it already.

Oh yes, I was a charmer. I also used to hold my breath if I didn't get what I wanted. I know, sounds like Congress, I may have missed my calling. But again, the seventies were a bit more relaxed. My pediatrician's advice was to let me pass out. My mom was appropriately aghast, even then, but he said "Oh, she won't actually pass out, her body won't let it get that far." HA! Listen, I may not have a lot, but I have got an outrageous stubborn streak. Which is why I dropped to the sidewalk one day due to lightheadedness due to holding my breath. I can't remember what I wanted so badly, but it was the last time I held my breath to get it.

My stubbornness didn't show up as early in my children, but we did have our share of early scares. Like when my eight-week old son caught a cold. I'm not being sarcastic or implying anything about overly protective parents – I'm talking about a cold that turned into a hospital stay. Congratulations, you now have something new to worry about. You're welcome. My son had a cold that seemed to be getting into his chest, so my pediatrician advised us to watch out for Bronchiolitis. This delightful event would signal its arrival by the "sucking in" of his lungs.

"If his lungs suck in, take him to the ER."

"OK, what does that look like?"

"You'll know it when you see it."

Hmmm… that doesn't bode well. Fast forward forty-eight hours and I'm giving the little guy a bath when all of a sudden I realize—his lungs are sucking in. The doc wasn't kidding, this is not easy to describe, but essentially it looked like the skin and top of his stomach was being pulled up and under his rib cage with every breath. As if a hand was inside his body grabbed his stomach and yanked, pulling the skin and muscles of his stomach up and underneath his rib cage. Technically it was his diaphragm, I guess, but no matter the part, it sure as poop did not look comfortable and it absolutely did not look normal. A quick consult and we were off to the Emergency Room.

I've spent a bit of time in Emergency Rooms but this was different. Emergency Room for me? No problem. Emergency Room for my child? No thank you. It is very, very difficult to watch procedures happen that you know are hurting your kid, but are absolutely necessary. Just seeing an IV put into my sons' tiny arm was enough to send me over the edge, so my heart bleeds for parents dealing with so much worse. I arrived at the ER, demanded attention Sorry, child who was there with an actual life-threatening allergic reaction, Mama Bear was in charge of my decisions.

An eight-week-old is not who they want to see in an ER, and the response was immediate. As described in my other book, the doctor was speaking with me, so I knew things were OK. Had he ignored me entirely and focused on my son, that's a worry. There were things for him to inhale and things to attach and things to monitor. And an excellent, decades long conversation about why I needed a breast pump at that moment then. No, I didn't think to bring it with me. Given that it took the better part of two hours to get one I probably could have driven home and gotten it. And no, he couldn't nurse at the time, he was attached to this that and the other and had a nebulizer mask over his face. As he screamed. You know what? I don't owe you an explanation. I needed a breast pump because I needed a breast pump. Fine. If you can't imagine why I had to nurse or pump RIGHT THEN, let me help. Imagine filling a balloon until it's ready to burst but it doesn't stop filling, it just gets more and more painfully full. Yes, that's why breasts of nursing moms sometimes leak. So they don't explode. But honestly, my exploding breasts were the least of my problems or would have been if I didn't have to keep explaining to the professionals calling the maternity ward why I needed a breast pump. Yes! Right now! Oh, who cares, just get me a pad or something to sop this mess up. None of this matters, my son is in safe hands, and he and I got to spend the night up on the pediatric ward.

Our family has a habit of being the youngest patient in any given ward. I was once trapped for four days on the cardiac floor at the tender age of forty-four. He was fine, though. He actually fell asleep during the doctor's exam the next morning. We left the hospital, I panicked every seven and a half minutes or so for the next week, even brought him back to the ER because he seemed worse to me. That trip was fun, I knew I'd overreacted as soon as we got there, don't care check him anyway please, he's eight weeks old. I got to listen to two doctors, the attending and someone new to the rotation discussing the eight-week-old baby's lungs right outside our curtain. Essentially the 'oh man you gotta hear this' conversation. And then the new doc came in, with some BS about "just need to check, just a routine thing..." I let him create what I'm sure he thought was a very solid sounding medical reason for him to be there, and then asked, "So you want to hear the eight-week old's crackling lungs, right? Not your typical patient?" He wasn't even sheepish, which I respected. "Go right ahead." Hey, if listening to my kids' lungs for two seconds when it isn't medically necessary is going to help you diagnose someone in the future, go for it. Hospitals are really one giant experiment – only the doctors are the mice and we are the maze. Help a little critter out if you can, there's a lot of different kinds of cheese.

Luckily not all injuries are life threatening. I spent my entire childhood with two Band-Aids over my knees. I distinctly recall peeling off one to uncover a scab of pretty decent thickness. Who could wait long enough for healed skin? I then revealed the other scab, same deal. Unfortunately, I did this while riding my bike, which shortly necessitated the addition of more Band-Aids. And not every trip to the ER is a crisis, of course. Some are just absurd. I was traveling with my daughter pretty regularly back to the east coast. I had a small production company, and we would go for a month at a time to get a show started or do a training or a festival. Anyway, we often shared a bed. My daughter was around four and into pony beads, which are little smooth plastic beads that are the exact size of the opening in your ear. You'll know it when you see one. Or feel one.

So, back to a lovely Sunday morning, I was just coming to and my daughter was trying to wake me by tickling my face. Not unusual for her, and also not unusual that as a toddler the concept of tickling, i.e., 'touching lightly to make someone laugh,' was not grasped in its entirety. She was smacking my face and head.

"Tickle tickle!"

"Oh honey, please, just give mommy five minutes. If you want to tickle someone, you just barely touch them. Like a butterfly. Not a tank."

"OK Mama."

And I drifted off again. I woke to my ear being tickled. Huh. She figured it out. I rolled over to say good morning, but it felt like her finger was still on my ear.

"Wait, what... honey what is in my ear?"

"A bead."

"A bee?"

"No a bead, a beaD."

A bead. Is in my ear. I immediately tilted my head and did a little shake. I knew high school swim team would come in handy one day. Nope, didn't work. I shook, banged, twisted, rattled— nothing. I ran to the bathroom and using a contraption of two mirrors, several sticks of gum, a chopstick and the formula for static electricity and I could see... nada. Great. No idea what to do. It's Sunday morning. There's no other adult in the house, per my life, as it's a rental while I work on a show. No one around. And it's Sunday. No urgent care is open, nothing. Great. We're off to the ER. One hundred dollars. One hundred dollars to get that friggin' pony bead, which was a lovely bright yellow, by the way, out of my ear. It wasn't painful, it just wasn't a necessary part of my Sunday morning. And I wanted the doc to handle the teachable moment for me, so I asked him – please, tell my daughter why we can't put things in someone's ear. The medical explanation he launched into could have been a lecture for ENT specialists (Ear, Nose, Throat). Now, my girl is smart and she was at four, but this lecture was straight over her head. "You could have broken mommy's ear. BROKEN it. Thanks, doc, I'll take it from here."

Beads are tricky. Avoid beads. We had another one, a pretty green bead that caused a lot of trouble a few years later. My son found it and immediately put it to use. Not in his ear, mind you. In his nose. But only because we had a flight to catch. Any other day he'd have ignored it of course. And it wasn't just any bead, oh no it was a very round, very smooth, shiny bead with the smallest of pinholes. When you've been holding your son still for so long as they dig around in his nasal cavity trying to get a grip on a bead that fifteen minutes have passed and you can't feel your arms, so you have to tag team in your husband for the last five, it really makes twenty-three hours of labor. Look. Like. Nothing.

There will be problems. There will be doctors, there will be urgent care, there may even be hospitals. It will be OK. Scary things happen. You are not going to panic because you are the grownup. Focus on what you can do. Panicking never helps.

SUNNY SIDE UP

Surprise! You want to kill people. Parenting has been described as watching your heart walk around outside your body. Not by me, mind you, by someone poetic. I don't have time to refer to parenting in poetic ways because in the time it takes me to come up with a metaphor, my children get into fourteen fights over who was breathing too loud. Where was I? Ah, yes, violence.

I am a pacifist, have been for a quite a while. Once I realized there's an option between violence and non-violence, I leaned toward non-violence. It was not always this way. I got into at least three real fights when I was a young'n. The most memorable was a fight with a fourth grader who picked on my cousin. My cousin was both younger and smaller so of course I stepped in fists flying. I recall taking a book bag to my cheekbone. More specifically the corner of a book in the book bag to my cheekbone. By "taking" I mean he swung that thing around as hard as he could and smashed it into my face. Shockingly painful if I'm being honest. He really wound up. The parent in me thinks – ooh, teaching moment about centrifugal force. Thank god I didn't know me then. The physics of it all notwithstanding, I took my self-righteous self to his house and pounded on the door. "Look what your son did to me," I declared to his mom. She just stood there in a housedress and a confused expression. I glared at her for about a minute, got no response whatsoever, and left feeling I had done what I could do. There was no other parental involvement. I'm not recommending that; it's just how it was. As a grown up, well, I would make sure the child had his anger issues addressed. His anger issues, and the fact that he was kind of an asshole.

I also remember an absurd non-fight I got into with my next-door neighbor, a solidly built boy. His family was so exotic, his mom was Italian and his dad was Greek. I've no idea why that made them exotic; we were half Italian half Irish. I suspect it's because they ate different food, and I was picky in that "I've never seen that before I'm not eating it" kid way. My neighbor was two years younger, but he outweighed me by at least thirty pounds. It wasn't a real fight. It was more like a contest I was stupid enough to enter. The one where you say, "Let's punch each other in the stomach as hard as we can and see who wins." It's a testament to my early acting skills that I didn't retch right then all over him. Since that time, I've avoided actual violence pretty successfully. My pacifism isn't a political position, it's a fundamental philosophy. I assume that the humans I share the planet with do not want me punching, hitting scratching, maiming, harming, gutting, attacking, or blowing them up. This also applies to parts of their bodies and their family members.

Seems simple enough, violence and aggression, not a fan. And then my first child was born. And the mere thought, the fleeting, transient, random image of someone hurting her in the smallest of ways induced a red-hot rage haze that I've yet to recover from. Which is why my kids have to wear sunscreen. What? Bear with me. There are a thousand ways your kid can get hurt, and some of them you have to let happen. See *Finding Nemo*™ for more. Their hearts will be broken, either because they get their crush, or because their crush has no idea they exist. Or, because they find out at their fourteenth birthday party that The Crush took a walk with The Best Friend and they made out and it's not like you remember it like it was yesterday...

Wait, what are we talking about? Oh right, sunscreen.

Sunscreen is the hill I will die on. Given the state of the world, this might seem a small thing to focus on. Given the state of the world, I need to feel like I can accomplish something. Of all the heartbreak, world aches, bumps and bruises in my child's future, I had to focus on something I might actually be able to affect. Here's what I know – the sun isn't getting any cooler. The ozone isn't getting any thicker. Cancer isn't getting any kinder. And so – sunscreen. Of course, because it's the 21st century and everything, everything, everything can kill you, I know there are lists of ingredients and all kinds of things to be afraid of with sunscreen. Doesn't matter to me – we are lathering up, swimming in it, taking a good old bath in the sun screen. Because skin cancer. Pretty much preventable. I cannot protect you from everything, in fact I cannot protect you from most things, but I can attempt to keep your skin cells from attacking you. It's ain't much, but I feel like I've done something if I get sunscreen on the kids. Claim all the victories you can people. No small irony that it's a thin layer of protection I'm trying to impart. A bit of a shell against the onslaught of All That Out There. My dearest child, your friends may suck and the world may fall to pieces, but you won't have any suspicious moles. Not on my watch. Of course, all of this sun screen lathering may just be the extraterrestrial version of basting.

NIGHT BEFORE THE FIRST DAY OF SCHOOL MEDITATION

Deep breath...

Let her find her way around campus with ease,
And let him realize he needs the bathroom before he needs it.
Let her eat lunch with someone, preferably someone she likes,
And as a real bonus someone I think is a good influence but clearly that's asking too much for the first day so we'll just settle for not eating alone,
And let him be able to work the zipper on his lunch box. And his pants.
Let her have at least one class she likes,
And let him have a teacher who understands play is learning.
Let the school be safe.
Let the school be safe.
Let the school be safe.
And return them to my arms at the end of the day and somehow make it to bedtime without any of us collapsing.
And in return I will get up tomorrow and gladly do it all over again.

SAFETY

Defined *noun* The state of being safe; freedom from the occurrence of injury, risk or loss. *Antonym:* Alive.

PAIN defined: *noun P*hysical suffering or distress. Mental suffering or distress. The mental and physical suffering a parent undergoes when their child feels suffering or distress. An annoying or troublesome person or thing. *See siblings*

SAFETY FIRST

My track record is not the best when it comes to personal safety. My childhood didn't include walk-in urgent care because it didn't exist. There were no after hours options except the emergency room and that was for car accidents and heart attacks. The seventies were... different. Car beds instead of car seats, seat belts were rarely worn, bicycle helmets existed in the sense that sometimes kids like to ride bikes with cardboard boxes on their heads (no eye holes mind you) and playgrounds were built on a patch of hard dirt (zero cost) or a cement slab (fancy). How the hell did anyone survive? We are the reason for the helmet laws and the playground safety ideas.

I did my share of safety research for all of you. You're welcome! Fell off a playground apparatus to the cement when I was around four. I think. As you can imagine the memory is a wee bit fuzzy. I remember the top, and I remember the bottom, and in between not so much. It was a fireman's pole type thing, a slide alternative. My nine year old sister slid down and then my seven year old brother slid down and then my four year old self did not quite slide down so much as fell down. I didn't realize they were holding on as they slid so I didn't. I didn't hold on and I didn't slide. I hit the ground and I was immediately taken home, probably had an ice pack on my head. No permanent damage done as far as we know. My point was the apparatus was on a cement slab. My point was not how uncoordinated I was, although that is true, as I also fell off a short wall in front of my aunt's house onto the cement sidewalk. Again, probably around three or four years old. That time I blacked out and woke up on a couch with all my cousins staring at me. My uncle was a dentist, so that somehow qualified him to diagnose me and I was pronounced just fine. I believe I had a cold washcloth on my head for a while. Of course, these were my very active cousins, and someone had a cast on something at all times. At the time of my wall dive there was a thick plaster bandage across my cousin's busted nose. Earlier in the week he caught a golf club at the end of its swing with his face. Driving ranges are fun. His brother did it, but you really can't blame him. It's hard to swing a golf club wearing an arm sling and a cast. Where were we? Ah, safety precautions.

Presumably safety has been tossed out the window by someone, what with the existence of a baby and the endlessly euphemistic term 'safe sex' being what it is. Honestly, it's as if the only way anything can go wrong during sex is if someone gets pregnant. Seems like an exceptionally male point of view, if I'm being sexist myself. And I am. Speaking of sexism and danger, it's fun to play along sometimes and pretend I know how to cook or that I give a shit about learning. There I am in the kitchen, puttering around waving various utensils, burners going. It's probably no coincidence that I had a stroke while making breakfast. The universe saying, hey, you don't belong in here. While pregnant, though, there was nothing to blame but the baby brain. Baby brain is a phenomenon that has no scientific backing but happens to virtually every pregnant woman. Intelligent, sophisticated, world dominating women suddenly find themselves with access to only parts of their brain for intermittent periods of time. This is not to pretend that pregnant women shouldn't be in charge of things – we all know a woman with a half a brain is still light years ahead of the game. I don't know, maybe that's sexist. You can take that up with me as soon as you solve Equal Pay. *Hint to get you started: Equal pay is easy, because of what the word equal implies, i.e., the same. Equal pay doesn't require explanations, equivocations, or justifications. It's just equal.*

We're going to move on because that may take you a while to solve. The United States has been actively working on it since I was five years old and the result is NOT SO MUCH. For this next section, you can picture me in a frilly apron if it helps. My brain and I were in the kitchen, making rolls for dinner. By making I mean taking those little biscuits out of a blue nuclear waste tube and plopping them down on a baking sheet. Boom! Biscuits. Didn't matter, my belly was enormous so I was lucky I could even reach the stove. Biscuits into the oven at what, 350 degrees or so? Whatever. It was hot. I'm not taking credit for the stove – we were renting a flat at the time and 350 degrees could just have been 125 degrees or 475 degrees for all the stove knew. Ding! Time to take them out. All right, oven mitt or "cooking condom" on the left hand, pull those biscuits out, hand the tray off to my right hand and... My right hand. My right, extremely bare right hand is holding the extremely hot metal tray.

Because I am a woman and it was time for dinner, me, my hand and a bowl of ice went over to the table. I figured, eh, how bad can it be? Second degree burns are pretty bad, come to find out. Have you ever felt pain pulse with your heartbeat? It sounds like the title of a really bad techno dance song but in reality, it's worse. I described the pain to the ER admitting nurse as 'intermittent.' As in, outrageously painful, and then absolutely nothing. I believe, and have no science to back me up, that my nerves would overload then shutdown then repeat. It's fun to be pregnant and in pain because they can't give you anything much. I left with a topical to prevent infection. Which was a real consideration, given that all of my fingertips, the skin from forefinger to thumb and a good piece of my palm were scorched. Shoulda worn a condom.

THE STUPIDEST THING WE EVER DID

I'm told all the time that being a kid today is so much more dangerous than my childhood. The difference in growing up in the seventies wasn't that it wasn't dangerous. Just that the danger was brought on entirely by ourselves. And it's not that there isn't reason to fear for kids today. After all, we were all kids and we all did stupid things. How do I know? Because I did stupid things. I'm going to share a few of those now, which may reassure you or it may terrify you. Either way, stupid things done by moi. Yes, I devoted an entire chapter to this in an earlier book. Turns out there are more!

We lived in a neighborhood that was just two streets with a little connector, sometime after my town stopped being rural and before it fully succumbed to suburbia. You could drive down my street, loop up to Good Street, and back to Main St. That's it. Around thirty houses, all built in the fifties. Behind the neighborhood were the Seven Fields. As a child, the Seven Fields offered a range of possibilities that included not only the fields themselves, but also the Junk Yard, The Hill, The Swamp and other areas worthy of capital letters. We'd run through the First Field, past The Hill, down a long path to The Oak Tree and then, across another field, or maybe two (we really lost track of the numbering system at this point)- there was the Junk Yard. A still life of lost debris. I recall hunks and curling strips of metal, crumbly to the touch, all covered in powdery rust. And I remember getting in serious trouble for being back there – not because it was a junk yard and the potential for slicing ourselves open or getting stuck in a fridge was real, but because we had walked too far. But that wasn't the stupidest thing we did.

During the winter, there was The Hill (well I assume The Hill was there in the summer too, but at that point it was just a path to the junkyard, so we never noticed it). We sprinted through First Field to The Hill. The hill ended in a deep tree line, with a single skinny path continuing through the trees into The Swamp. And by skinny path, I mean maybe a few inches clearance on either side of the sled. So of course, that's where we headed. The goal was to start at the very top of the hill, gain maximum speed and then pray that you could thread the needle onto the path between the trees. And if you didn't, there were two options. Chicken out early, everyone diving off in a flying scramble of bodies, hats, boots and screams, or slam into one of the trees and then fall out in a scramble of bodies, hats, boots and screams. I probably should have mentioned that the minimum number of riders was three. Six to fourteen was preferred. And if you made it onto the path, you had the added bonus of then being in the middle of The Swamp. It wasn't an actual swamp; it was a marsh with a lot of elm trees in the midst. Hang on… turns out that is the definition of a swamp. So, added bonus of landing yourself in The Swamp, an actual real life swamp. You had to tread carefully, because whatever there was of ice covering the mushy marsh, and you could easily put a boot through it. And of course, there were alligators waiting under the ice. Waiting under the ice, in New England, in a freshwater marsh. Uh, YEAH! Why, are you saying there weren't? I pity your childhood. And yet. That wasn't the stupidest thing we did.

Winter also meant hockey. In the northeast, in the seventies, if you had on skates, you were playing hockey. What was the point of anything else? Half of us didn't even have hockey sticks, didn't matter, we'd be out there skating, oh, I don't know, interference? Nobody knew, nobody cared. We were outside, and we were playing hockey. We played in the street. No, not street hockey, although that was great; at a certain point in the winter the streets had been plowed so many times that a few inches of ice formed on top and you could skate on the street. This was before science ruined all street ice hockey opportunities by salting the roads. Harrumph. So not street hockey, I'm talking about river hockey. Not pond hockey, because it was definitely a river. We used the open, rounded part of it, right after one of the bridges. The river was wonderful. We weren't allowed to swim in it, but hockey was A-OK. We tore through the First Field and carried our skates to a certain point in The Swamp, a treeless area that was the start of a stream that led to the river. We sat in the snow, put our skates on, broke a lace, tried again and we were off. A quick skate down the little creek to the wide river to play hockey. Of course, it was The River mind you, so the freezing part was never fully cooperative. We often played "over here" because "over there" was open, unfrozen water. "Over here," white ice with a layer of snow on it we had to shovel off before we could play, "over there" gray ice slowly thinning the further you went until it was open black water. There were no sideboards there were no painted lines there were no edges or stop measures between us and the unfrozen, open black water. And even so, this was not the stupidest thing we did.

Have you noticed how we ran through the First Field? Always, always, always ran through the First Field. Would you like to know why? Because of Farmer Dodd's Wife. Farmer Dodd's wife was the wife of Farmer Dodd, presumably. We never met Farmer Dodd. No one did. I'm not sure he was even alive at that point. The farm was not being farmed, but it was used to grow hay and once a year the hay was rolled into enormous round bails which today would make the greatest paintball arena on earth. But back then, no. We ran through that field. Why? Farmer Dodd's Wife. Or more accurately, Farmer Dodd's Wife's Rifle. Yes, Farmer Dodd's Wife sat in the hayloft of their barn, looking out the window with a clear view of Field One and the top of The Hill (which is why running through Field One was often followed by diving over the ridge of The Hill). At any rate, she sat there, with a clear view and a loaded shotgun, waiting to shoot kids who came through her property. I nearly pissed myself when I had to knock on their door to sell Girl Scout cookies, let me tell you.

We had to steel ourselves to make the run. We huddled near the back of the Thompsons, right next to the wild grape bushes (at least, I hope they were wild grapes, we ate them) and then when the tension was too high to stand we took off as fast as we could, cleared the top of The Hill by hurling ourselves over it—and we were free to roam. Well, what's so stupid about that? It's smart to run through a field when someone has a rifle. Oh, that's not the stupid part. The stupid part is, coming home, we walked through First Field. Just strolled on through. For some unknown, kid logic reason, she was never waiting for us on the way home. Like she's sitting there, "Ah, those kids are so clever, forget it, I'll shoot 'em another day." I'm sure Mrs. Dodd (hey, maybe that was her name!) was very nice and I've no idea how the story started because I'm sure she didn't deserve it. But she gave us a hell of a lot more fun this way. And even this, this sauntering through a field with what I firmly believed was a rifle trained on my head because of neighborhood legend, this was not the stupidest thing we did.

Notice how none of these stories have adults in them? Except for Mrs. Dodd of course and she was trying to kill us. The stupidest thing we did was done with the full permission and sanction of the adults in our world.

"Ride without seatbelts?"

"Well, yes, we did that too, but that's not—"

"Sit with your feet hanging out the back of the station wagon as it drove around town?"

"Well yes, but that's not—"

"Voted to allow companies to market directly to children?"

"What??"

Yeah, that happened in the seventies, but the adults did that on their own. You probably don't remember, but it's the day the toy aisle exploded into the blue side and the pink side. Oh, OK, here it is: The stupidest thing we ever did was walk home in a blizzard. That is neither metaphor nor hyperbole.

You know the joke: when I was a kid, I walked ten miles to school, uphill, both ways, in a snowstorm. Did it. Swear to God. It was the winter of 1978 and New England was hit with what is creatively referred to as the Blizzard of '78. I was in elementary school, probably third grade, maybe fourth. I walked to school, about a mile. We cut through our neighborhood, crossed the high school parking lots, crossed the athletic fields behind the high school, through a little wood and there we were. One street away from school. In the winter, I wore a full snow suit, boots, hat, gloves, scarf, every conceivable piece of outerwear. My teacher called 'the walkers' to the front of the class a half hour before school ended to start helping us dress for the long campaign home. On this particular day, school let out early. The blizzard was already in full swing and they had to get the buses off the roads before they were closed. It was very exciting, everyone was thrilled, YAY no school today (we wouldn't be back for two weeks). Everyone bundled up, they put the kids on the buses in a rush – the roads were really getting treacherous. And they let us go. The walkers. Just let us walk out, into the blizzard, and trusted that we'd get home safely.

Walking was fine while we were on school property, because there were bright yellow buses going by, so it's not like we couldn't' tell where the road was (assuming they were on the road. That blizzard had more than three feet of snow and twenty-foot snow drifts. Seriously - stranded motorists, was blamed for more than one hundred deaths and did more than $520 million in damage. But go ahead kiddos, walk home!). Onward we walked. And we crossed the street just fine and got through the little copse of trees.

And then the problem hit. We came out of the woods and were face to face with... nothing. Absolutely nothing. A complete white out. We couldn't see the far side of the field; we couldn't see the little fence twenty feet in front of us. The school itself, a two-story structure that stretched a good quarter mile end to end – gone. Complete whiteout. Did we turn around, go back to school, insist that a grownup actually find us a safe way home? Nope. We were too stupid to go back, but at least we were smart enough to know that we couldn't set out across that field of nothing. The building was somewhere to our right, so we headed in that direction until we ran into it. And then we hugged it, creeping close around every corner and edge (it had been built in phases, patchwork like), kept going, going, past the doors that were near the cafeteria, past the locker room doors, still going, still zero visibility, past classroom windows all the way to the very last corner of the building. Nothing left but a long, sloping hill and then the parking lot. The wide, empty parking lot. Full of snow drifts. Maybe. Hold a piece of white paper about a half inch in front of your face. Ta da! You're in a blizzard white out. Perhaps stand in your freezer if you'd like the full effect. So what did we do? Well, it was cold, and nobody wanted to wait, and nobody was going to try and go back, so we just walked. Walked straight out into that mess and kept going.

~

I DON'T KNOW how we made it to the street on the far side, it was down a little hill but who could tell with the snow drifts. I don't think we even knew we had crossed the street until we hit the Devon's red fence, maybe fifty feet back from the road. Followed that along to Mr. McClean's hedge, followed that to the end of his property, climbed a few snow drifts as we crossed what might have been the street and walked until we bumped into my house. Which is where I left the group. No idea if those other kids ever made it home. Turns out we got thirty to forty inches of snow that day, and three thousand cars were abandoned on the highway. No one ever said a word about how dangerous it must have been for us to walk home; we just didn't consider it. So the stupidest thing we did was trust the adults who said it was OK to go home. The truth is, none of us know what the hell we're doing, and we're the grownups now.

THE TOY THAT MUST NOT BE NAMED

There are many trials of parenthood designed to test not only your patience, but also your strength and your ability to withstand pain. These include but are not limited to nursing a child with teeth, cute little pudgy fingers grasping a fistful of hair (chest, head, beard, whatever) and giving it a good yank, and stepping barefoot on a Lego which may rank with the pain of childbirth. Not really but we'll throw the dudes a bone. And then, there is the most dangerous, I dare say evil toy on the market.

Glitter.

Glitter is evil.

Glitter is the opposite of creativity. When I want something to look like I don't know how to be creative, I add glitter.

Oh, I know what you're thinking, glitter is not a toy. Ha! I say, and again I say Ha! So that would be Ha Ha! You see, glitter may not be a toy in the traditional sense, but it is most certainly a toy in the sense of evoking a wonder and rapture that can only be rivaled I assume, by drugs. I wouldn't know. It starts out innocent. It may not even happen at home. Maybe your child is in a carefully researched preschool and they put a little glitter on an art project. That doesn't seem so bad. Until you realize that one thumbprint of glitter translates into a tsunami of sparkle invading your house. Oh, it doesn't even matter if your kid actually likes glitter. The glitter is coming, and it is unstoppable. It may appear to be stuck to the art project, it may appear to be innocently gleaming, a bit of sparkle. If it hasn't shown up before, I promise you it will appear in a St. Patrick's Day Homage to Rainbows and Legends of Green People and It. Will. Suck. That's right. Because once it shows up, you can't get rid of it. Once it shows up, it stays forever. But, but but my kid doesn't like glitter! My kid won't do that! We've got a carefully researched and developed art and self expression dynamic in our home. We have an art cart, an art corner, a full blown art studio, my kid has seen Michelangelo's *The David* for crying out loud in person in Florence and not been kicked out for accidentally taking pictures with a flash like some people. Apologies, I digress. That may have been me. You don't have to believe me. You can sit there in denial.

"Oh, not *my* kid. My kid won't do glitter. My kid WON'T do glitter."

"Oh, but he will."

"No. NO. First of all, he's a boy."

That might buy you a little time, gender politics being what they are, but eventually, eventually, he's coming home with a project covered in glitter. And it all seems fine. It sparkles, it's kind of pretty, there are different colors. Hope you like them. Hope you really, really like them.

Because they aren't going anywhere.

You'll be picking it out of your rug (we have hardwoods) then you'll be picking it out of your dog's hair (we have a hairless cat) then you'll be picking it out of your kid's noses, if they haven't gotten to it themselves. Because it never goes away. Oh come on, what's a little glitter? What's the worst thing that can happen? A little extra sparkle in the house, that sounds great. Uh huh. We won't discuss the fact (true and scientifically proven, if those words still mean anything when this is published) that there is now so much glitter in the world that it is showing up in fish. In. Fish. That's right – little Nemo and big ole Moby Dick are swimming around in so many tiny plastic particles that they are ingesting them in measurable amounts and the Rainbow Fish story has come to life in the most horrifying way. Good heavens.

"How many pots of gold do you need Timmy? Huh? HUH? Answer me- do you want Dory to die? Oh, I didn't mean- no it's OK."

Well, it's not OK. Glitter fish may not even be the worst part. No, that's absurd, that is the worst part but I have more to say. Think about what you lose. What you give up for glitter. Where maybe a nice swirl of paint, or some kind of drawing would take place – uh uh. Nope. Glitter. Perhaps a photo over here, or a little description or even a one word label – NO! G-l-i-t-t-e-r. Fight it. Fight it as hard as you can. Because one day, your kids' English teacher will have to instruct twelfth graders that their research paper does not, I repeat, does not require glitter. And the disappointment in the room will be palpable.

"But but but Miss, how will we know it's a project if we don't put glitter on it?"

"Your project will answer the thesis question, that's how you'll know you've done a good job. Not by the trail of sparkles you leave behind you, nor the snow globe environment you create while dropping said project on my desk."

"Are you sure?"

I'm sure. I'm absolutely certain. Whatever you do, don't do glitter.

Glitter: The gateway drug to a lack of creativity. Like crack for kids.

GROSS

Defined: *adjective* Disgusting, lacking in refinement or good manners, without deductions, total amount of sales. *Before children, the couple enjoyed their entire paycheck, or gross income.*

NO THANKS, S'NOT FOR ME

Everyone is obsessed with body parts, even the aliens. What do you think all that probing is about? Chances are, you have some body parts. Your baby might as well. There may be some male parts, there may be some female parts, but in general, what you've given birth to is a human. It's important to keep this in mind. There are entire industries devoted to making you forget that you are raising a human being. It's far better for them if you are willing to clarify with great pride, "I'm raising a boy human" or "I'm raising a girl human." This increases profits by, well, double. I'm no business expert, but twice as much is definitely more. Around two times more, give or take.

In the beginning, the body parts are simple, because it's really both ends and the general coziness that you are dealing with. Feeding, pooping, temperature regulation and sleeping all directly related to the body parts. Of course, you've likely been concerned from the beginning with body parts, what with the ultrasounds and all. In fact, you may have found out early which particular body parts your little human will have. And if you did, good for you. Whatever that means for you – good for you. I'm not entirely sure how the preparations differ, but it seems like some people find it more fun that way, and we're all for fun over here in the Basso house. Where was I? Ah, yes, body parts.

There are some excellent aspects of new human bodies. First, they are adorable. Not immediately, and not as a whole. Immediately after birth, humans resemble nothing so much as a little alien, covered in goo, in some shade of pink, blue, purple, grey or a startling combination thereof. Definitely the cooler end of the spectrum. Yellow is a color you want to avoid, but even that one isn't unusual. There may be hair, there may not be hair. There may be hair in unexpected places. No matter. Your little alien arrived. Oh, excuse me. Your baby, and I mean this sincerely, is the cutest thing in the world as was mine. It's all those other babies, if we're being honest, that are not all that cute. Yeah, sorry. I don't actually believe that, I think tiny toes and tiny noses are adorbs to use an annoyingly shortened word. But show a picture of a newborn covered in goo to a child and they say, "Ew." Which is honest.

And then the snot comes. I'm not a squeamish person, I've dealt with some pretty overwhelming diapers with great calm. I've dealt with whatever that stuff is I'm growing in the back of the fridge. But nose mucous is my limit. Yeah, the occasional little booger is cute, but the full sneeze mouth and chin covered in slime? No. No way. Oh, I'll help. I'll grab forty tissues and press them against that little face and wipe repeatedly. But I'd prefer to be wearing a hazmat suit. That's just me.

I amend my earlier statement – you have the food going in hole, the food coming out hole and the nose hole. When I was young and adorable, I called my nose the place where the 'God Bless You's' come out. How charming! As if slime and muck is a delightful little gift from above. I was referring at the time, to the two tiny black triangles on my Raggedy Ann's larger red triangle of a nose. I just realized Raggedy Ann is part jack o'lantern. Interesting.

The fun really rolls when your little person discovers their own body parts. Toes and nose and oh my that grows. This is a joyful time – because these toys have already been paid for, they are always with you, they don't run on batteries, and frankly there's a lot of exploration that needs to happen, best get navigating. You may try to limit it to the bedroom, or your home. Timmy's penis is great fun for him, but do you want him sharing that joy on the playground? Probably not.

You will of course have an intimate understanding of your alien's digestive system, as there's no limits on where, when, or how your new human defecates. Go ahead and celebrate in the beginning, everyone does because it's great to know the parts work. Those joys will multiply in the weeks, months, nay years to come. As will the smells whenever a new food is introduced. So many smells. So very many smells. It's a lot of joy. Almost overwhelming. Gag worthy in fact. Though it seems impossible, the day will come when your child will, more or less, use the toilet. At some point, you will no longer be responsible for diapering. This in no way implies that you are no longer responsible for urine and poop. In fact, this is the equivalent of raising a condor in captivity for release later – you are merely setting the feces free in the hope that it finds its proper place in the world. Commonly, the toilet. Before we leave diapering, let's take a look back at some of the highlights…

POOP. YOURS, THE BABY'S, AND THE CAT'S, OR OH SHIT.

It seems appropriate that the word poop is spelled the same frontwards and backwards; it is after all, endless. An extended part of your day, nay your life, will be a never-ending attempt to clean your child's bottom. You keep feeding them, they will keep making poop. True story. So, congratulations parent! Poop is now an integral part of your life. Not that it hasn't been up to now; I certainly hope you haven't been holding it in.

Understand – you are responsible for cleaning all areas of poop. No, no, listen closely. I said "areas of poop." Not "you are responsible for changing diapers." All. Areas. Of. Poop. If you recall from sixth grade, area is the length times the width times the depth times a billion. Plus whatever the dog dragged around. The baby is going to pee on you. Thank the baby when this happens. It's going to get so much worse. Also, understand, your baby can fart louder that you can. Don't get into a contest, you will lose. In the world of competitive farting, your baby is a sonic boom, and you are a gentle breeze.

In the beginning, there was poop. In the middle, there was poop. And of course, the end is full of... poop.

Lest we devolve into poor bathroom humor, I've devised a glossary, nay, a compendium of poop propers so we can all pretend we're grownups with college degrees and mortgages and that we are not simply wiping some mammal's ass all day long. A mammal that we love of course (yeah, I felt you judging me). I give you:

THE POOP LEXICON

Up the Back Poop – A tidal wave of poop that smears up the entire back surface of your baby until it laps at her hair. Advanced babies will include the splash zone, which is a sophisticated around the hip maneuver, and back down into the diaper, leaving every possible nook and cranny coated. Belly buttons are cute until they are filled with feces. Bonus points for ears. This is not to be confused with Back Splash Poop, or Lick It Ridge, in which a ridge of poop appears above the diaper line in the back. You may not be able to catch this, sightings are rare, because the dog will likely eat it before you get to it.

Rainbow Poop -Bonus points if you can identify any of it.

Baby Food Poop - identifiable only in that it's color and texture defy description

Poop that Might Not Be Poop, But Since It's in the Diaper We'll Call It That Anyway- This usually happens around the time your genius learns how to shove things in her diaper. Could be anything. Food. Toys. The cat. The cat litter. Rocks. Caterpillars. This will immediately trigger real poop, thereby coating this little surprise in fecal goodness.

Growth Spurt Poop- If your genius is sitting in his highchair and is suddenly 3 inches taller don't call the NBA. There is simply a giant and potentially hard poop lying in wait. Of course, if he sinks back down immediately this could be morphing into an up the back poop, and you'll want to act fast.

HALLELUJAH POOP- When the digestive system decides to get moving again after a week and a half. More common than you think.

A LAST WORD ON POOP, also known as advice for you to ignore: If you don't have a dog, get one immediately, as soon as you find out you are pregnant. Get as young a dog as possible. Not only will this give you much needed practice in picking up poop in unexpected places, but the dog will graduate to rummaging through the garbage (and or diaper pail) and spreading the contents for all to share after the baby is born. Because nothing is as fun as slipping on a dirty diaper and landing in a pile of shredded poop!

ARE YOU GONNA EAT THAT?

Don't think things are all hunky dory at the other end of the digestive system. There are problems there as well. I don't recommend even reading this bit if you are having any kind of pregnancy related nausea like morning sickness, parent related nausea like other parents judging you, or author related nausea, caused by that last section on poop.

The good news is that all of these treats are already part of the cooking you regularly do. The bad news is, they represent your new "I Must be the Mom/Dad" menu.

RECIPES FOR MOM-IFIED TASTE BUDS*

Day Old Everything

Oh Dear God I Don't Think that's Chocolate

Burnt *including*:

- Burnt on the edges but still good
- Completely burnt
- Burnt on the outside, undercooked on the inside

- And its antithesis: Oh Shit I Forgot to Turn on the Stove. Again.

Leftovers *including*:

- Chicken, or what the FDA passes for chicken in that last mega-nugget left on your kid's plate.
- This Half of this Piece of Lettuce isn't Rotten
- I Don't Think This is Supposed to be Yogurt
- Look at That – New Mushrooms!
- We Really Should Have Labeled This (from the back of the fridge)

Frozen Leftovers *including*:

- Square block of Something in a Square Shaped Container
- Rectangular Block of Something in a Rectangular Container
- Undisclosed Shape Encased in Extremely Wrinkled Tin Foil – Proceed with Caution

And don't forget your Fruits and Veggies:

- Broccoli Stems
- The Brown Banana
- The Weird Looking Carrot

Bon Appetit!

*I argued with myself for ten minutes over well to say Parent-ified instead of Mom-ified and then I realized I don't know a single man who eats this way.

CLEAN

Defined *adjective* Free from dirt* unstained** unsoiled***

*OK, that's possible eventually

**Also possible with great effort

***Give me a break. If you children are going to play, at all, things are going to be soiled, broken, busted and otherwise destroyed

CLEANLINESS IS NEXT TO...

IMPOSSIBLE

My sister and I shared a room, but we didn't need a line of tape down the middle to divide the property. Her side of the room had a regularly scheduled laundry day for her dolls' clothes. My side had a regularly scheduled chewing out from our mother. Even now my piles of papers seem to self-propagate. Currently, I am responsible not only for my own cleanliness but for the cleanliness of other humans. Fortunately science proved that excessive cleanliness contributes to the strains of super bugs currently destroying our immune system. In the name of science and your well-being, I have donated the interior of my car and most of my house. You're welcome.

In our house, my car is whatever car my husband is has finished driving. Sounds like a gender issue but here's the truth - I don't care what I drive. I need to go from here to there and I'm not super concerned with the trappings, apart from gas mileage. I also don't care for car payments. Those are particularly annoying, given that I'm supposed to pay them every flipping month at the same time. So. Cars. Not a high standard over here, but even I find my kids' treatment of the car abhorrent. They're like a couple of drunks in the bar bathroom. Whatever it was didn't leak out the door? Success! Doesn't matter if there is a garbage can in the vehicle, a trash container of some kind, that banana peel is still going to find its way under the seat, where it will petrify into a dense, fibrous steel cable fused to the floor panel. Even so, it's like tenth on the list of glue-like substances that are either near or coming out of your child. Your car, someone else's car, doesn't matter. While traveling with my three year old daughter, we returned our borrowed car and startled dismantling the car seat for the flight home. Ah, the unchartered delights that await you under the car seat. I suggest leaving it in place the entirety of your alien's childhood to maximize the super virus fighting properties (see above). In our case, today's treasure was a distinctly waxy substance covering the back seat. My nose, so adept at distinguishing au de child aromas locked onto the distinct odor and rainbow of colors du jour.

"What's this?"

"K-ons."

"Crayons? We didn't bring any crayons when did you get crayons?"

"Da store."

"You bought crayons without my knowledge?

"The food store."

"The food store? You stole crayons from a grocery store?"

"No no no. Mama. Listen my words. The K-ons wit da macncheese."

"Oh."

Damn you, helpful restaurant with your child's placemat. Three half stubs of crayon turned into a river of wax, given the right temperature and the ticking clock of a waiting flight home. Oh, I know, there's a thousand quick fix hacks out there, but when you're trying to catch a plane, you just don't have time to rifle through all the easy DIY heart surgery hacks and the never need another light bulb remedies to find a way to remove wax from upholstery using a solar panel and double sided tape. We were in that car for about four minutes, by the way.

On the other hand, my childhood car was spotless, but that's only because you can't eat, draw, or make a mess when you're holding on for dear life as you bounce around without a seat belt.

#REALISH

Let me be clear – I think Mommy Blogs are great. True, I am not a fan of "lifestyles," mainly because I don't know what that means – isn't the style in which we live our lives our lifestyle? And isn't it a lifestyle whether or not anything matches? Perhaps, perhaps not. That's for the influencers to figure out. At any rate, I prefer a life to a lifestyle, if I have to choose. No matter though – because I do love Mommy Blogs.

If you're not familiar, a Mommy Blog is where a mom has gorgeously lit photos of her family and home that essentially show you everything you could do to improve your family's life which has the potential to make you feel bad but it's written in such a way that it makes you feel good because the blogger is relentlessly, unswervingly, undeniably supportive. But that's not why I like them. I like them, because for once, moms are gaming the system. That's right. You know that eight million bazillion dollar industry that is parenthood? Well, Mommy Bloggers have worked out how to get the products they need and show off their sweet managerial skills at the same time. It's smart. It's profitable (I hope). And it's helpful, to them and to other parents looking for ideas. It's just not real.

You know how I know when a mommy blog, at least one that pretends to be real life, is full of bananas? It's not the lack of surprise vomit or the sparkling empty sinks. It's the lack of boogers. That's right, not a booger to be found. I'm not suggesting it. I have seen parents post videos of their kids pooping. I feel like the kid should have a say if they want their bowel movements televised. Remarkably, though, no boogers. Likewise, there's no dust. No detritus. Sure, the floor is cluttered with toys that were quite possibly staged (or maybe my kids are the only ones who don't have color coordinated play time) but the floor itself is clean. CLEAN. I know, because if you look at the edge of the rug, there's no backup of random things. Come to think of it, the area rug is lying smoothly on the floor, squared off to the wall. Because the dice, cars, hair doodles and leftover graham crackers aren't making little bumps in it and the dogs didn't just slide into it and crumple it against the wall. Again. Amateurs.

All I'm saying is, totally cool that you're pretending you know what a cluttered house looks like, but unless the dust is acting like an accidental filter for your camera – you've got some catching up to do. You're gonna have to let it go, probably for several months, if you want to compete with this action. Oh, I know, you put a hashtag on it that says "real" but yeah. Not buying it. Also, the simple fact that it's a camera means you're editing what we see, because you're pointing the lens. Hey, your blog, your call. And I genuinely love a well framed shot. But it's not real.

You want to get real? Give your kid permission to have a social account in which she is allowed to take pics of your pets and only your pets and see how that goes. I'll tell you – you think you're safe, but she'll manage to photograph them not only sitting on a dirty floor, while lounging on a pile of dirty laundry, the angle of the shot will include every dust bunny you have (we fondly refer to them as dust capybaras over here because they tend to be quite large). She'll also manage to include your bra in several shots and what could quite possibly be a sanitary napkin removed from the trash. If you aren't familiar with how cats feel about used pads and tampons, do not get a cat. They are first and foremost carnivores. That's all I'm saying. Feel like you're ready to bare it all? Get real and keep it real for the masses? Give the camera to your kid and let the social anxiety slide over you like an icy blanket. That, my friends, is #reallife.

WHY I DON'T WANT MY KIDS AFRAID OF WORDS

OR HOW I JUSTIFY CURSING SO MUCH

Clean also often refers to language. Not in our house, but in others. I've seen it- honest to goodness adults saying, "Oh jiminy snicker doodles, that really burns my butter bonnet." A child is born, and an adult becomes a poor version of Dr. Seuss, "Oh karsniffler frick-ity fracker!" Or so I'm told. I get it, I do. Everyone has their thing, their battle, and for some people it's "I will not swear and my children will not swear and all will be right with the world." I understand. We have to pick our battles. Yours, perhaps, is cursing. Here's why mine isn't.

While it's true that I would love for my children to speak eloquently on a variety of subjects and respond to even the most difficult of situations with aplomb and verve, the truth is, I don't want them to be afraid of anything, most of all, words. I have not always cursed like a sailor. My parents, in fact, were adamant that cursing was a near unforgivable event. This in spite of the fact that my father cursed with great gusto and regularity, particularly in the car. "Are you shitting me?" is an honest to goodness phrase in Boston, to which my dad would reply, "Do you feel like you're falling?"

Hypocrisy aside, there were words kids are allowed to use, and there were words grownups are allowed to use. It was always tricky. I remember when I learned my first curse word. Well, technically, I learned how to spell it. My brother and I were talking and he asked me if I knew how to spell jerk. What forbidden fruit is this? And then he told me, "G-E-R-K." For a long time, I thought gherkins were somehow naughty pickles, and if there's not a hidden innuendo there than I don't know my pickles.

Yes. Jerk was my first curse word. We weren't allowed to call each other names. I know. It seems so quaint. We also weren't allowed to say that we hated people. Being Roman Catholic, and excessively so, I was taught that to say I hated someone meant that, given the opportunity and the proper connections, I would damn them to hell for all eternity, or until the cable guy showed up, whichever came first. Cable was yet to be invented so eternity it was! My parents were serious about this. I remember a neighborhood friend, who regularly told his mom he hated her. I decided to try it out one day. The first of many errors regarding where to draw the line. I was told to sit on the couch and wait for my father to come home. Oh dear god. Like waiting to vomit, waiting for my father to come home was infinitely worse than whatever punishment was coming. Never clever enough to mess up late in the afternoon, my waits were sometimes quite lengthy.

Of course, there was always the wooden spoon option. Oh yes. The wooden spoon came out for a quick rap on my backside, nothing permanent, nothing actually damaging. Unless you count the fact that I can't hear a squeaky drawer without diving under the table. No, I'm kidding. About the diving, not the squeak. Because of course the wooden spoon was kept in the drawer with the other cooking utensils, and of course it had an awful squeak. While mom was making dinner we were all in a constant panic. The drawer squeaked open "He did it" and shut, "Whew."

So. There was good reason not to curse. But the variety and scope of words available was almost too much to keep up with, and only got worse as I aged. We all know that there are no fewer than 3,458 terms for the word vagina, but the one that got me was- vagina. I swear. I was so used to hearing euphemisms and acronyms and slang and other words that are not terms for vagina. Quick, how many can you think of? My husband has a catalog of thousands. Most of them disgusting, some quite hilarious, rarely adorable. So there I am, in sixth grade, and I hear the word vagina for the first time. I thought it was a made up word. Vagina? Are you kidding? Are you trying to say Virginia? What are you talking about? Thus began my quest that my children would know the proper term for things. And that has grown to include people who are assholes.

I curse freely and without reservation in the privacy of my own home. Accidentally, I curse in public no more than nine or ten times a day. My cat is regularly referred to as a shit bird. She is. She is a true flight of poop sailing through our lives, with random attacks and evil ambushes awaiting our every move. I come from a long line of door slammers and cupboard bangers and others who are not afraid to make some noise. We're Italian. Subtlety is not a concern. Our dining room table growing up was incredibly loud – everyone had something to say, everyone had an opinion, everyone was talking over everyone. It was wonderful. And we were full participants as kids, we never sat quietly, we had things to say and we said them, and my parents listened. I've always felt what I said was important (how could anyone be a writer otherwise?) and I have my parents to thank for that. The self-inflated ego that went with it, well, that interpretation of my brilliance is entirely on my shoulders.

I truly don't want my kids to be afraid of words. I don't want someone to be able to say something to them and have the choice of words make them respond as if they are under attack. They may be under attack, but they are under attack from the person, not the words. It's a subtle difference but I feel like it makes a world of difference. When someone uses a word, let's say bitch, because that's still probably the most socially acceptable term to call a woman (if I used the word c*nt here half of you might stop reading and need to get a glass of water. In fact, just seeing three of the four letters in that word can make people woozy.) The attempt is obviously to diminish the woman being spoken to. It's a weak desperate move—a focus on the big bad word so the person can hide. No one with a justifiable argument ever called their opponent a name. Or mocked them. Not since PreK. Nothing says "I don't have an argument" like resorting to name calling and mockery. And if you don't agree with me, you're a poo-poo head.

My kids curse, I'm sure of it. Or if they don't now, they will. Point of fact, they know subtleties of grammar, colloquial usage, hell they could teach a master class. These curses are nouns, these are verbs, and this one, ah this one is the everything all-purpose every part of speech wonder child. Amen. And I'm fine with that. Because someday, someone's going to call them a ______ and they won't bat an eye. They'll understand, of course, the level of diminishment that person is trying to lay on them. My personal favorite is "shut up" which is not in fact a curse word, but a complete denial of the other human being. And my response of course, is always to keep talking. If you want me to shut up, you're going to have to have a compelling argument for me to do so. Otherwise, you are going to be in it until you run from the room or you puncture your own eardrums with a fork. Shut up is like, please step on the gas pedal, I need to know Everything You Are Thinking.

The best curses, of course, smite your enemies. I had the good fortune to stay in a little mountain village in Italy, and the people I met were exceptionally specific with their curses, i.e., "may a sack of slightly mold potatoes with four to seven eyes each fall on your head from a great height." Your status as a parent gives you untold reams of power in this regard. Someone I know hates me, because the following curses have been used on me to great effect:

May your child wet the bed. Yours.
May you walk barefoot on a sea of Legos.
May you pull the last diaper from the bag as you board the plane.

May your child projectile vomit. From the top bunk.

My mother's version of this was more personal, but so subtle. She'd regularly tell me:

I hope you have seven just like you.

And I'd stomp off to my room thinking, "I will, I will have seven just like me and at least I'll understand them and it will be great SO THERE!" It didn't happen. My kids are nothing like me. Sure, my teen spends an exceptional amount of time writing books and telling me I'm wrong and my son considers putting something away landing it in the general area of his room but... Oh.

PLURPLE

Never will the extraterrestrial nature of your child be more evident than when spoken language begins. Up to this point, your little one has to some degree resembled other humanistic forms. Not so with language. Otherworldly screams and babbles. Or perhaps, a complete lack of verbiage. I suspect these children are of vastly superior intelligence and have realized early on that there may or may not be intelligent life here. That or they're waiting until they have something to say. Walking and talking can happen around roughly the same time. And they say (you know, "they" the ones with all the answers) that a kid can do one or the other but it's really hard to develop both simultaneously. Seems unfair. Maybe that's why kids wail when they drop on their butts for the nineteenth time during a three-step walk, it's not that it hurts to land on a diaper padded butt it's simply they don't have the vocabulary to express frustration. And their parents are saying things like, "Oh diddly doo, you dropped on your bummy-kins." I'd scream too.

Verbal communication can be difficult at any age, clearly. I traveled to Italy shortly after breaking my pinkie finger. I don't recall how. How I broke my finger, I mean. I do remember I traveled via Italian Air and that I vividly recall because of the great food and handsome Italian flight attendants. Even at twenty-one I could recognize a pack of silver foxes. The accent didn't hurt. I also recall the brace on my poor broken digit, which was crushed by every Italian I met, enthusiastically pumping the hand of the American with the strangely oversized ring on her little finger. What they accepted as fashion from me simply did not translate:

"Broken, my finger is broken."

"So you decorated it? Have something to eat."

It's disconcerting to know how truly stupid the rest of the world thinks we are. And that was in 1991. I stayed with a family on that trip that was French and Italian and you'd think the linguistic possibilities for their kids would double. Turned out they tripled. Their house spoke Italian, French, and whatever the hell the toddler was saying. The oldest child was bilingual by five and very intelligent thank goodness, because it turns out she needed to be trilingual. She had to translate for her little brother. To the rest of us he sounded like "le le le la, la la le, le le le lalala. La." To be honest, much of French sounds like that to me anyway, seeing as I don't speak French. Or Italian for that matter. Or English, if I'm having a stroke. But that was just that one time so it's fine.

You can be sure when the time came Lovely Hubby and I never did the "ba ba" for bottle thing – I figure it's tough enough for the little alien to learn a language, why make them learn it twice? Not that it matters much either way. For the first three to seven years of life, much of what your child says will be intelligible only to you. My toddler's translations have nothing to do with your toddler's translations. Using my translations would be like using a Spanish dictionary to try to speak Mandarin with a person who speaks only German. Each toddler is a linguistic island unto themselves. Good luck! I'll wait here while you work that out.

All set? Great. Once you've figured out what words are being said, you're about halfway there. Because now you have to figure out what the hell they mean. For example, when your toddler states, "I can do it myself" translations may include:

1. I can do it myself.
2. I can do it myself but I want you to watch me do it.
3. I can do it myself but only if you aren't looking.
4. I can do it myself but I want you and everyone within a five mile radius to watch me do it.
5. Do it for me.
6. Do it for me but don't let me know you're doing it for me.
7. I'm going to do it myself even though I don't know what it is or what I'm doing with it.
8. I need a nap.
9. I'm hungry.
10. I've now been insisting on doing this myself for so long I've forgotten what it is that I'm doing but I'm certain I can in fact do it myself and if you come anywhere near me I'll be aggravated at a level the likes of which have never been seen.

Note: It's possible for all these translations to be accurate at the same time. That's called a tantrum. There's a teenager version of this that is identical, but with a more pronounced sheen of confusion on everything and the very real possibility it's being recorded or live-streamed.

LAZY

Defined: adjective Averse or disinclined to work, activity, or exertion. Or as I like to call it, efficient. *I am aversely disinclined to clean up after you.*

also See Author photo

note The discussion of lazy will be brief for obvious reasons.

LAZY! GIVE ME AN L! GIVE ME AN...

OH NEVERMIND

Lazy. I am a lazy parent. Absolutely, one hundred percent. I don't mean I'm not involved; I am, I volunteer left right and center. But when it comes to actually doing things for my children? Lazy. Let's justify that shall we?

Ah dear dear Lazy. You've treated me well. If the section on cleanliness didn't convince you, allow me to describe myself in a word. It's that one at the top of the page do I have to say it again? I once sat in a mommy meeting—I know, that's hard to picture. Other parents subjected to this in person. Your empathy speaks well of you. I had no choice and neither did they. My son was enrolled in a co-operative pre-school with parenting classes as part of the curriculum. We all sat down once a week and gave great advice to each other. It was wonderful. Until the day we talked about choosing between the daily grind of chores and playing with your kids.

"Given the choice, do you do chores or play with your kids?"

Me: "Play."

Everyone else: "Chores. "

Me: "Wait, what?"

I listened as grownups, parents I admired, lamented the fact that they would love to play a game with their littles or snuggle up on the couch and have some movie time, but they had to get those dishes done. Really? Why? It literally doesn't occur to me to get the dishes done (yes, yes, woe is Lovely Hubby. I have other skills, he's fine). I mean, it occurs to me, but given the chance, I'll take snuggle time any time. No question. Let the damn dishes pile up honestly, no one ever said, I wish I did more dishes.

My aversion to doing things I don't have to do started young. One of my chores as a child was to bring everyone's laundry upstairs. The rest of the family sauntered by their neatly folded (not by me) laundry and went on up. Excuse me, couldn't you just take it on the way? Nope. That's your job. I was also asked to dry dishes. There is literally no point in drying a dish. The air, which is free and readily available, will do it for you. True story. Likewise, there is no reason to wash a child's face. The dog, who is free (if you adopt a mutt) and readily available, will do it for you. I also became a director almost immediately upon entering the theater industry – why would I do all that acting over and over and over; I'll direct and get other people to tell the story for me. Duh. And they seem to enjoy doing it, so win-win! Imagine my confusion as a teacher when a parent contacted me to negotiate their child's grade. High school student mind you, though I find this absurd at any age, given that grades in elementary school are meaningless. Don't tell my youngest. So Concerned Mom of a Twelfth Grader called me to discuss the grade, as if the grade the child had earned wasn't the grade the child had earned. I went on at length as you can imagine:

"I'd like to talk about Joe Joe's grade. You gave him a C."

"No, he earned a C."

Time passes, grass grows.

"Anything else?"

You can imagine my aversion to effort when it comes to parenting. I mean, you'll have to obviously. It's not like I'm going to do it. The moment, the absolute moment my children figure out how to do something – they own it. At seven months my son was stealing food from my plate. Great! You fix dinner. I'll be over here.

Is there more?

Nah, that covers it.

MAMA

Defined: *noun* See previous chapters

Mama Bear: If you have to ask, it's already too late

WILD KINGDOM

Sure, the idea of someone hurting your child can bring out the rage in any of us. But Mama Bear instincts notwithstanding, we don't really have much in common with the average bear. Protecting our young, yes, but there's an entire planet of beings out there raising young without the use of books, hospitals or opposable thumbs. After all, it's a rare lion seen propping up a parenting manual while trying to take down a gazelle single pawed. Or triple pawed, I guess, what with the four legs. My childhood was filled with wild animals, and not just those of us roaming the neighborhood in packs. Every Sunday night, at 7pm, Mutual of Omaha presented Wild Kingdom. Yes, I am old enough to know TV shows that were presented by specific companies. Presumably Mutual of Omaha did a bangin' business in wildlife insurance policies. This is less funny now that I live in a town regularly visited by mountain lions in a state regularly ravaged by drought in a country regularly confused by the need for clean air and water in a world on fire. It's OK, though because aliens love s'mores as much as we do.

"Mom, my human isn't toasting correctly!"

"Put it back into the fire. No, not the oil fire in the Gulf, the natural fires in California. We eat organic!"

No such confusion in the animal kingdom of course, they understand the need for clean air, clean water. That's why they get it bottled and driven in on a truck. The show mainly consisted of lions eating gazelles, tigers eating gazelles, armies of fire ants eating gazelles. Gazelles getting drunk to stave off the horror of their impending doom. Oh, and lions having sex. I definitely remember that one. They just kept at it until there was a young'un or two. And some even worked together to raise them. In general, animals also don't judge the parenting skills of others, though some do steal their neighbor's offspring. For dinner.

I am somewhat less carnivorous than the average lion, though I do feel a kinship, a connection to these creatures sharing the planet with us. Like most people, my spirit animal is a sea horse. For those of you less spiritual and more Harry Potter minded, my Patronus, of course, is a giraffe. Slightly less common and rather difficult to get going out the end of the wand (giraffes are notoriously lazy magical beings) but worth it in the end for sheer spectacle. And while I readily admit that we humans are the top of the food chain, I don't necessarily believe we are the most intelligent beings in it. I suspect there's a cephalopod somewhere just waiting for us to destroy ourselves, so she can rule in peace and benevolence. I digress.

I know the basics about giraffes but not a thing about their parenting skills. My delight in them is really based on their unusual physicality. The neck, the coat. Giraffes after all are one of a kind. Flamingos come close, with their equally graceful necks. But a giraffe is a skyscraper of an animal. Competing with trees. No one ever asked a giraffe if she thought heels would look better. And sea horses – absolutely absurd in their vertical alignment, tiny fins, randomly curling tail. Don't get me started on the ones that look like dragons. Too late! Adorable! Almost enough to get me to want to write fantasy. Until I remember I suck at directions so I'd never be able to make the requisite map for the end papers. My authorship failings to the side, I wondered if my spirit animals might have some parenting advice to offer. I've never seen a sea horse, or a giraffe for that matter, take advice from a stranger in a grocery store, so clearly, they've something to tell.

First of all, they tell us we are extremely lucky. The average baby giraffe is six feet tall, and that's not the hard part. They weigh between one hundred and one hundred fifty pounds. That's the baby, not mom. That's a lot of neck. And a lot of legs, come to think of it. Also, that baby giraffe is hanging out in there for fifteen months, a full half year longer than we instant gratification humans. Being born a baby giraffe is no picnic either – and I mean the actual process of being born. Yeah, I know, it's not fun for any of us, what with the squishing of the head and the shock of cold air and all. But at least someone catches you! That's right – giraffes have their young while standing up so that tangle of neck and legs hits the ground from six feet in the air. Boom! Welcome to the world, here's some dirt on your tongue. From a medical standpoint, this drop-in style serves many purposes, not the least of which is the umbilical cord is severed and therefore the young giraffe is 'encouraged' to take its first breaths. Encouragement like gasping, "Holy crap what the hell just happened?" and "Where did the floor go?" and the somewhat less popular "I didn't get to finish my crossword puzzle!" I imagine some newborn, legs akimbo, lying there asking, "Am I breathing? Mom, is this breathing? Is this how you do it?" It's an interesting idea. Could save on medical costs. Nope, doc you don't need to be there to catch, we're going to let gravity take care of that. Yikes.

Standing is encouraged shortly thereafter. Again, extremely different from our approach. Because if you want to nurse from a mama giraffe, you're going to have to pick yourself up out of the dirt. Standing and walking are highly applauded skills from an early age. Your child is not a giraffe, and there are no lions chasing her. So, chill on the teach 'em to walk stuff, honestly, mobility just means it's unlikely you'll be able to hide from your kid.

As for the actual parenting, giraffes have a distinct advantage over humans in that they rarely sleep. On purpose. Sorry: giraffes rarely sleep on purpose. Forgot to add that in there. In the wild, giraffes are looking at anywhere from thirty minute to a few hours in any 24-hour period. Again, this is because the lions are salivating nearby. Still, no giraffe is scrambling to find a coffee substitute that actually works like caffeine because she's nursing. In fact, the young are often hidden for hours at a time because they can't keep up with the grazing herd. I'm not suggesting you stash your kid somewhere and disappear. Though I believe that's called Grandma's.

And my other favorite, the sea horse? Come on, what's the one thing you know about seahorses? Say it with me:

They're too small to ride.

No, no of course not. The males take care of the young. There's really nothing else to say, except try to get some "me time" male seahorses. In the unlikely event that you aren't feeling either of these choices, please flip to the "Find Your Parenting Spirit Animal" feature.

FIND YOUR PARENTING SPIRIT ANIMAL

Welcome to the interactive portion of the book. When the aliens arrive (the rest of them, I mean, I assume my people are coming), we won't be the only species they check out. Why not get a head start, and possibly find your parenting style from this handy dandy barely scientific list to boot?[1]

Are you a turtle? Do you tend to go for large numbers of offspring and wander off for a swim after giving birth? Do you have an inexplicable desire to give birth in moonlight on a beach? By the way if this birthing movement doesn't already exist, I'm patenting it. Just saying. Going to call it Hump Moms. No, Moms with Leathernecks. Ah, I have it: Moonlight Mamas. Everyone is doing it. How else are you going to get sand in your vagina?

Are you a seal? Do you spend eleven months pregnant? Like, that kid is hanging out in there forever? Not saying I blame them; I mean as a seal the average temp in your neighborhood hovers around 'freeze your knickers off' degrees. Are you the type to toss that kid at two weeks old into freezing water for swim lessons? Presumably to get back at them for the extended gestation. Again, no blame. Do you do this every single year, year in and year out, without the help of the father? You may in fact already be a seal. No one seems to know where the male seals are. Bermuda one assumes.

If you're deeply into homeschooling, you may be an orangutan. One child every nine years, eight of which are spent in intensive homeschooling including agricultural studies (gathering fruit) and advanced engineering and home repair (nest building). Must be very comfortable with heights. Very comfortable. Like spend all your time in the trees Lorax comfortable.

Are you a Caecilian parent? It doesn't matter because their parenting style is as disgusting as they look, and you should not pick this one. They are not charmers. Imagine the juiciest, slickest looking worm you can think of, and make it up to five feet long. Only it isn't a worm, it's an amphibian. The adorable offspring lick nutrients off of mom – and – get this – eat her skin. Yup. EAT HER SKIN. It has a lot of good fat; plus, every few days she grows more skin to keep the buffet going. Heaven help us. Just the idea of this, I'm trying to put on moisturizer, the kids are snacking on me, it's too much. I know, I know, I said I wouldn't judge but I forbid you to do this. I forbid it. Stop talking. It's not happening. No.

Do you run your house like a game show episode created by Darwin? Do you disagree with everything I said in that section about competition? Hello, my pushy friend the Lace Wing Spider. Oh, you're pushy. A little too pushy for your own good. That's right, you push your kids. Literally shove your kids into an attack, triggering their cannibal instinct to eat you. It's one way to get out of car pool. But I'm not sure on the logistics, do you wait until their first set of teeth are in? Their second set? Do you want to be gnawed by adorable little TicTac teeth or shredded by full grown canines? It's a lot to take in. I do however, completely understand the "oh screw it" aspect of this. Just give up. Fine. FINE! Eat me. Whatever. At least I can nap.

Hold on... turns out a lot of moms get eaten by their kids, which is a great metaphor for the need for self-care. Take care of yourself, because someday your kids may need to eat you. Mother Nature knows everything. Great. Any parents who don't get eaten? Are there any dads involved? Oh, absolutely, and not just the aforementioned sea horse. Have a look:

HAS THE SIBLING RIVALRY IN YOUR HOUSE GOTTEN A LITTLE OUT OF HAND? Are your kids trying to eat each other? You could be a very cute, very poisonous tree frog. Does your parenting process begin with the daddy guarding the kids/eggs and peeing on them? Clearly not! But since your little human will be peeing all over you we'll just call it even. The tadpoles arrive seriously pissed off and ready to kill, I can only assume because they've been peed on. But since they need pops to help feed them, they turn on their siblings. Dad worked way too hard peeing on those kids to have them just devour each other, so every child gets its own room. Way up in the trees, their own private little dewdrop swimming pool, and who has to manage this fantastic solution to sibling rivalry? Mom does. Dad had to pee on them, and Mom delivers an unfertilized egg every damn day to more than fifty kids all over that flipping tree. The human equivalent of this daily trek is a separate apartment for each child at opposite ends of town. Honestly. This is why we eat at the dining room table isn't it? To contain the mess to one room? And the ceiling. And that little bit of the hallway. Someone find the dog to lick this up. No, don't hold the dog up to the ceiling. Forget it. I'll be at an apartment across town.

LOVING PREGNANCY AND WISH IT COULD GO ON FOREVER OR TWENTY-FOUR MONTHS WHICHEVER COMES FIRST? Want to give birth every few years well into your seventies? Congratulations, you're an elephant. Of course, you also rule the herd, and bring up your young in a group of like-minded badass women. For example, you go after other herds who elephant-nap one of your own. Which implies that some elephants they also kidnap kids from other groups. So, let's see, that's a kid every two years until you're seventy... plus your kids have kids every two years... carry the five... math still sucks by the way... That's a lot of children and grand-children, plus some additional kids what with the elephant-napping. I'm not saying don't do it, I'm just saying, I don't think there's a lot of time to relax.

Maybe your kids haven't eaten you, but have you forgotten to eat? Did you give birth to one hundred thousand children simultaneously at the bottom of the ocean? Yup, that's a huge brood, Madame Octopus, one and done well done you. BAM. No time for self-care. But don't worry, it doesn't last long. After six months of round the clock nurturing and utter starvation on your part, you'll have the chance to watch an adorable school play called "We're All Hatching" and die mid-clap. The end thanks so much.

Are you terrified yet? See? I told you this book would make you feel better about parenting. Parenting a human, I mean. If you want to know what it's like to parent an alien, you'll have to ask my parents.

BACKYARD KINGDOM

The animal kingdom can be a dangerous and horrifying place to look for parenting advice. If you don't believe me, read the preceding section. There is a slightly less wild, more common animal often used for parenting practice – the average mutt. And in a lot of ways it's a great idea. A baby, like a dog, is a living being that must be fed, watered, and not abandoned when it stops being cute or chews up the carpet. Like babies and parents, dogs and dog owners have been sucked into a maelstrom of food, toy, and comfort items befitting a mega-industry. I was going to get an actual number for that, but there's no point because it grows exponentially every day. So certainly, a fur baby is good practice. Many would argue that a fur baby is enough – no need for the kiddos. But if you are serious about parenting prep, there's a better option.

Gardening. Yes, I know, those tomatoes aren't going to lick your face the way a Labrador would and they'll never be part of the family. Particularly since the plan is to eat them. But for the sheer unknowingness of parenting, the cliff drop of hope and a prayer, the never-ending experiment of unknown variables called parenting, gardening is most apt. More akin to parenting in terms of the patience, work, and overall attentiveness required, and the benefits of benign neglect. Benign neglect, mind you, not actual neglect. You don't need to agree, I'm not that fragile, but let's walk through this.

First, there's a seed. It goes in the soil, you know it's there; you know something is happening, but you can't see it. That's pregnancy. Sure, we have ultrasounds and way to listen in on the proceedings and an excellent idea of how it all works, but we don't actually witness it bit by bit. Probably why everyone is so obsessed with the size of the growth at each stage of pregnancy. First it's a seed, then a grape, then a peach, then an eggplant, then a salad bar... At some point, you can tell from the outside that something is going on. And I should hope so. Not a fan of the "I got pregnant and I didn't gain any weight/pretend modest giggle" BS thing that was happening a few years ago. You're supposed to gain weight. You're growing a person. Point of fact, the increased blood supply alone needed to adequately nourish a fetus can be around four pounds.

At any rate, in your garden, finally, a tender green shoot arrives. Tada! Birthday for the tomato. It's thrilling, and terrifying, because now other things can see it too. Things that are not as in love with it as you are, things that in fact may harm it, or in the case of my garden, kill it outright. I have never despised a snail so much as when I found it munching on a tender pea leaf. And when I pulled it off, that little creep held on, ripped that little pea flower right off with it. Not quite Mama Bear rage, but close. My actual children of course rescued the snail, painted its shell, put it in a bucket and fed it my best tomato. Children are awful stick to plants.

But beware, just like kids, seeds have minds of their own. I've planted things in the fall that were supposed to sprout in three weeks. Six months later, after a rare, heavy rainfall, they decided it was time. I couldn't rush that. I couldn't force that. No one ever talked a seed into using the potty. Flash cards won't help a green bean. Know what I mean? Just, you know, don't eat your kids.

~

My mom is an exceptional gardener, her thumb a deep forest green. The growing season in New England is short, just a few months, but she packed the veggies into our garden and like everyone, they listened to her. Summertime chores included picking a salad for dinner. I loved the picking, hated the eating. I still consider veggies homework. Mom also coaxed four hundred peaches out of a single tree and let me tell you the fun we did not have spending days in a hot humid kitchen canning peaches.

Nowadays there's a movement back to home gardening so kids will know their food didn't arrive on the planet in a plastic bag with a price tag. Or at least that the fries come from a genetically modified starch globule and not a fry fairy.

Seventies parents weren't looking for teachable moments, their kids time was spent outside "until the streetlights came on." Sum total of parental involvement in our after-school activities was the demand to "be home by the time the streetlights come on." I don't know how those streetlights knew when we needed to be back, but I assumed my mom had an in with the government. And it was a great outdoors to be in; changing seasons, different sports to play. Lots of trees for climbing. We had a weeping willow that let us play under her skirts, a perfectly round room, secret and special. Our absolute best tree was a huge three-kids-can't-connect-arms-around-it oak tree. Absolutely gorgeous, so we attacked it with hammers and odd bits of wood and built a magnificent double decker tree house with trap doors and wall-to-wall carpeting made of carpet samples. Pretty slick. Up the ladder, through the trap door into the first floor. And then the second-floor access was out a window and onto a roof. I'm fairly sure the roof, I mean second story, wouldn't pass inspection as an actual floor but kid construction rarely gets permitted. At least in those days. Today I hear people build tree houses for the kids, which seems pointless. How are you going to learn to use a hammer if you don't smash your thumb a few thousand times? Also, how is it "yours" if you didn't build it? I'm telling you, that tree house with its ladder made of mismatched wood was a real point of pride. My parents certainly weren't going to slam their shins on that one rung that was worn slippery smooth and yet somehow gave us massive splinters at the same time. They don't manufacture them like that you have to dig in the junkyard for that kind of thing.

Smashed thumbs and shins aside, there was occasionally a slight danger in using the products of Kids, Inc. The time a friend fell out of the Tree House and split her chin open on a rock eight feet below. Technically not the Tree House's fault, it did add an air of mystique and murder to the proceedings. For years, that bloodstained rock withstood snowstorms and thundershowers to warn us all. We gathered around it like ants, small in the face of its majesty. But like ACME on the Saturday morning cartoons, the quality of our products didn't seem to matter, the customers kept coming. We once built a bike jump specifically for bikes with five or more people on them that failed miserably. Or, spectacularly if we're getting points for the number of broken bones. The point is, being outside is good for kids. Maybe not in an 'avoid urgent care' kind of way, but I'm sure there's some benefit.

We were pretty outdoorsy in general, mainly because my mom and dad were obsessed with yard work, particularly the length of the grass. As a child, I firmly believed the purpose of children was to mow their parent's lawns, where I now know the purpose of children is to do my dishes. In a truly inspired moment, my folks planted a tree for each of us in our yard. My sister, the eldest, a flowering cherry. Lovely. My brother, the only boy, an elm. Stately, elegant. And then I was born. The youngest, clearly the most revered and cherished child. They planted a crab apple tree. Wait, what? There's an excruciatingly awkward photo of me around fifth grade with a pixie cut, a 'Here Comes Trouble' tee shirt and a smile to make an orthodontist drool standing in front of that crab apple tree. I tried really hard to find it for this book. In my thirteenth year, we had a rare New England hurricane. Our trees were okay. At first. Until the wind lifted the skirts of the huge weeping willow, flipped her over, and smashed her onto my tree. My tree, planted when I was born, crushed at thirteen years old. Good thing I'm not superstitious.

Death omens notwithstanding, your own backyard offers excellent models for parenting. But again, don't eat the children.

ENOUGH

Defined*: adjective* Adequate. And that's enough of that.

NO*: adverb Negative,* used to express denial, refusal, dissent

Nooooooooo!: *exclamation* used to express denial, anguish and pain, often seen at dinner and bedtime.

No no no no NO! *exclamation* often seen when markers are introduced to a child

No. Absolutely Not! *declarative* used when tween inquires when she will be getting her navel pierced

No way what the hell?!? *rhetorical question* used when teen arrives home with navel pierced

SUMMERTIME AND THE LIVING IS HUMID

A childhood summer should be idyllic, filled with lazy days and swims in the swimming hole. Or so a certain series of books on the prairie told me. Our little house, while darling, was 180 degrees from Memorial Day through Labor Day, and there was no AC. Not even a window unit. We used to sleep on the screened in porch just to combat the sweats and the tangle of drenched sheets. Very *To Kill a Mockingbird.*

My parents had an ongoing battle of wills called "the house is too hot what should we do?" Mom volleyed first, as she marched into our rooms at the crack of dawn, snapping the shades up and shouting "Good morning Sunshine" to the other weirdos happy to be awake before noon. And then she'd throw the windows open to boot, in spite of the 271% humidity that is a New England summer. Very bath house. Very take a shower and never be able to dry off. Very bleh. And Dad marched along behind her, muttering random words I was never supposed to say and shutting the windows when she wasn't looking. At some point between dripping sweat and passing out, Mom noticed the closed windows. Cue a twenty minute discussion of "we need to open the windows for a cross breeze no we don't we should keep everything closed tightly to try and keep the house cool." Dad had physics on his side but logic was no match for my mother. This is a woman who once threw out an entire set of encyclopedias because they were old. So presumably the information was expired. Oh, yes, the family mocked her, right up until the Internet put encyclopedias out of business.

"Why on earth did you throw out the encyclopedias?

"They're old!"

"So the information expired?"

Well the jokes on us and we all owe her a heartfelt apology. Not it!

We dripped our way through a decade or so, and then Dad put the ceiling fan in the hallway. We did all our own house projects. It was a great way to spend seven times the time and eighty times the stress. The ceiling fan took a record one day to install, and only one more day to flip and then just one more for the electrical and really Bill let's just open the windows for a cross breeze. This magnificent fan, my father assured us, would draw the hot air out of the bedrooms, into the attic and out of the house. Once we installed the whirly bird on the roof.

"So, like a cross breeze," we said.

He grounded us.

The fan was spectacularly huge, like a jet engine. And just as quiet.

I remember being so happy to go to bed that night thinking we'd finally cool off. My father waited for everyone to be in bed, heads flipped towards the door to, yes, you got it, feel the cross breeze. The sound started low, barely noticeable. And as the rumble built, and built, the whole house began to tremble and the curtains went slightly, well they went horizontal. Hands grabbed onto bedframes as legs lifted airborne. We held onto our beds for dear life. We weren't any cooler, because the wind was still 120 degrees, and we had to dodge lighter objects like books and dressers pulled into the maelstrom, but no one noticed. Too busy surviving the cross breeze.

Summer was filled with renovations like this, and I don't ever recall another person being there to help. There were small mishaps. My father, slicing off the tip of his finger while laying tile. He wrapped it in a maxi pad and kept going. Those things are absorbent, and this was before gel inserts. At some point a vacation was in order. Unfortunately, we didn't do vacations - we camped. There is a distinct difference between the two particularly in the days that tents weighed upwards of ninety pounds and were made of canvas. My earliest memory is of camping – climbing up onto a rock next to my brother, near a little lake. Or probably a pond. My mom told me I was only a year old when we took that trip and couldn't possibly remember it. And yet, there it sits, in my memory, clear as day. No, there are no pictures of it. Didn't we cover this? Each family was allotted one roll of 24 exposures per camera per vacation, and it usually fell in the lake or was eaten by a raccoon.

Camping was cheap, even cheaper than now, and didn't even require a reservation. You just showed up, tossed down your tent, and hoped that the bathrooms weren't completely covered in spiders. If they were you hoped they had a working light so you could keep an eye on the spiders while you peed.

My parents also invented staycations in 1973. Prove it? Fine. Having no money to go anywhere, during the golden summer of my fourth year, my parents put in an in-ground pool. How is this possible in a family with no cash? Nothing exciting, we didn't DIY a pool out of milk cartons and coffee filters, we just kept it in the family. My uncle brought over a backhoe and dug out the hole and I'm fairly certain my other cousins poured the cement. I didn't ask why my Italian cousins had a cement truck and you shouldn't either. It was glorious. An in-ground pool. Probably fifteen feet by thirty feet, it had a deep end all of eight feet deep and oh heaven- a diving board. Which required skill to use and not slam your head into the bottom of the pool (again, only eight feet deep). We learned to swim young, because my dad was a former lifeguard. Point of fact, my dad has held every job in the known universe, up to and including rocket scientist. There isn't an industry, organization, or occupation mentioned in my father's presence that he hasn't participated in. Next time I see him I'm going to start talking prostitutes just to see what happens. Anyway, pops was a lifeguard, and mom was terrified of the water. My grandfather was terrified of the water, and therefore my mother terrified of the water. Fear is inheritable. Making matters worse, we all joined the swim team in high school. That had to suck. Come to think of it she did not attend swim meets.

We had a pool and no reason to go anywhere again. Vacations were held twenty feet out the backdoor, with the occasional side excursion to the front sidewalk to lay out our towels, bake on the hot cement and de-prune our fingers. To say life was simpler is to miss the point, we didn't have options. Day time TV was soap operas, and there was no such thing as cable. Cable. Cable? It's what happened before the Internet. It literally meant cable, oh never mind.

It was a simple set up and we knew we were lucky. First on our block to have a pool. Damn lucky. And my folks shared it widely with the neighborhood who spent most of that summer cooling off with us. Otherwise the river of sweat would have swept us all away. The problem was, some of our neighbors mistook us for an actual public pool. Oh, I don't mean pool hopping at night, everyone did that. This was… ruder. A woman we'll call Confused showed up one day to complain to the management of our pool. Namely my dad. Seems she was deeply disappointed in our level of service.

"My child is not getting adequate pool time."

"Ah, interesting," said my pops. I stuck around, popsicle dripping down my fingers. Even at four I knew that look. It was the look that said the battle over the cross breeze was going to look like flirting compared to this.

"In what way?" he continued, like a proper concierge. He probably was a concierge at some point but I was only four, so it hadn't come up. Yet.

"Well. My child is not getting the same amount of pool time as the other children, as I just said."

Pops smiled and gave her the good news.

"Well I have a solution for you. Your child will no longer be swimming in our pool. At all. Thanks for stopping by."

See that? Not only did my parents invent staycations, my dad was blocking people before Twitter ™ existed. Face to face.

NO IS THE ANSWER

All you need is... No.

No is an answer. For your kids, and for you. A wise woman once told me, "No is an answer. It is a complete sentence." Justification is not needed. Now, she was talking about the barrage of volunteer things parents are supposed to do (more on that elsewhere) but for me, No is also an answer for my children. And justification is not needed because logic is rarely at play in their requests.

"No, you cannot put the cat in the drawer. Again."

"No, you cannot pull out all the drawers and try to climb the dresser."

"No, you cannot draw on the dresser drawers with Sharpie. Or crayons. Or anything really."

"Yes! I am the worst mother in the world, thank you! Twenty points."

Sometimes they aren't old enough to understand the justification. Sometimes they just don't want to understand it and sometimes they are too busy slamming doors or rolling eyes to comprehend, well, anything. And sometimes, the world conspires against you. Like the ice cream truck. Never once has the ice cream truck shown up at a good time.

Ah, the ice cream truck. That harbinger of summer sweetness. As a child, it sent me flying to my dad's top drawer to rummage for change. My parents were not the type to just hand us a five and say have at it. Probably because ice cream cost a quarter and we had a minimum of both fives and quarters. For my children, the ice cream truck meant a jingle jangle song from a scratchy speaker at all hours of the night. And I do mean all hours – Lovely Hubby suspected the ice cream truck may have been dispensing something other than ice cream. Given that it was out at two a.m., it's possible. That jingle jangle, though, that song induces a craving, a desire, a need so deep it could carve marble. Of course, we told our children that the ice cream man only plays the song *when he's out of ice cream.* A tidbit I learned from another wise woman (it takes a Village People).

"Ooh, kids – hear the bells? Uh, oh, he must be out of ice cream. Telling everyone know there's no more today. Nice of him to let us know, right?"

Eventually this genius maneuver was thwarted by the ice cream truck just sitting there all day at the park. We got in the habit of picking up an ice cream cone on the way home. Or rather, a hyper-processed-over-colored-turn-your-poop-blue food coloring saturated dairy-ish treat. You know what I'm saying. Healthy. But a great way to bribe them off the playground. What that? Oh sure, you should never ever bribe your kids because oh I don't know some other book. The "children" or for our purposes "alien invaders" quickly learned that if they ran in opposite directions, I could only chase one of them at a time. When I caught the younger one in my arms, it slowed me down trying to catch the older one. So. Ice cream. Why not. On this particular day, my wallet was not with us. It happens. A lot. Or when I need to be conveniently out of cash.

"Well, kiddos, looks like no ice cream today."

"Oh no," the kind ice cream lady assured me, "Take two. I will be here again next time, I'm sure, just pay me then."

"No, it's OK."

The other parents were aghast. That giant sucking sound? Both an intake of breath and an exhalation of judgement. It takes practice.

"No, it's really fine. They'll be OK. No one ever died by not having an ice cream cone for once."

The other parents shielded their children's eyes, as we walked in shame, with no ice cream, to our car which we then drove to our house and our refrigerator of food really for the love of fuck is this actually a problem?

Mean lady. Probably. Oh well. My children lack for nothing in the food and nutrition area, so a missed treat is neither going to crush nor starve them. And it's not my job to make sure life is perfect – you know why? Because it simply isn't. It's my job is to go through life with you, and help you realize that life goes on even after disappointments, that sometimes it's necessary to be resilient, that you aren't always going to win and that's a good thing. Because if you don't like losing, you'll figure out a different way to win, or try a different thing.

Spoiler: My kids did not in fact die that day because they didn't get an ice cream. But they did learn to check my pockets for my wallet before we left the house.

"No" can also save a lot of pain and hassle in the teen years, but it needs to be a firm "No" like a real no like you say to the dog when they try to pee on the carpet. And it takes time to build that kind of stamina. I will admit this: I know, unequivocally, that as strict as my parents were, they saved me a lot of hassle. Some levels of teen stupidity (that other chapter on childhood stupidity doesn't count) were simply not an option for me. When I said, "I can't do that, because my parents will kill me" what I meant was, "I can't do that, because my parents will kill me." Being Catholic, there would not only be death but disappointment. Which was worse.

NEVER SAY NEVER

EXCEPT

1. Never assume your children are wearing shoes.
2. Never assume you removed all the stickers your toddler put on you. Specifically, the ones on your nipples. But they were smiley faces, so at least I know my breasts were happy. As do the ninety other people I passed today who didn't mention it.
3. When allowing a toddler to use chalk on your face as makeup, remember that it doesn't weigh anything, and it's very difficult to tell that it's still there. Again, no one will mention that you are a light shade of blue, like a no-budget remake of *Avatar*.
4. Never assume your children are wearing pants. Or that you have yours on the right way.
5. Never assume that because you handed your child a lunchbox and watched him put it in his backpack that it will still be there after walking twenty feet to the car.
6. Never assume that because your children have used the same seat in the car for years, what with their age appropriate car seats and all, that they won't argue over where to sit every day for two weeks, before suddenly deciding that where they sit is OK and instead have a knock down drag out fight over who gets to get into the car first.

7. Never assume that the answer "yes" to "did you brush your teeth?" means that teeth were brushed in recent memory. They may be referring to that time the dental hygienist scraped them like she was de-frosting a cake.
8. Never, ever, assume that your children are less capable than a top-notch law firm in the arts of plausible deniability, lies of omission and pleading the fifth all at the same time.

PRIVACY

Defined: *noun* Concealed from view, apart from other people, free from scrutiny. Including people at the grocery store. No longer an option.

ALONE WITH MY THOUGHTS

OR, SO YOU'RE SAYING SOLITARY CONFINEMENT IS NOT A VACATION? INTERESTING.

When I was very small, my mom worked at home. She was a medical transcriptionist. She wore headphones, pressed a pedal with her foot which started the tape rolling so she could listen to the doctor's diagnosis which she then typed while having a conversation with me about why she wouldn't let us add a third story to the tree house. No privacy whatsoever for her work. On the other hand, we were not allowed in my parents' bedroom without permission. And no one, absolutely no one would ever have even considered going into the bathroom when mom or dad was in there. Lovely Hubby and I have gone horribly wrong somewhere. When they say there's no privacy these days, because of social media and all, it confuses me. That's where I feel most alone, because my kid don't have accounts.

Picture a cozy family. Parent, child, maybe a dog. A hamster. A giraffe. Tidied up in a little house, so dear, so familiar. Got it? Good. Stay here as long as you like, because it's the last time you'll be alone with your thoughts.

You will never go to the bathroom alone again. I don't care how many bathrooms you have; I don't care how many times you move to a bigger house; I don't care if you are giving birth to a Royal. You will never go to the bathroom alone again. Never. Nope. No YOU listen: Never. I haven't gone to the bathroom alone in more than a decade. Not because I need help, but because that's the best time to ask me questions. I'm a captive audience, trapped on the toilet with nothing to do but solve sibling rivalry. For even when your offspring are able to go on their own, they will come and visit you, as you desperately scroll social media and pray those scary people who tapped into your phone are not secretly recording you while you defecate. But if they are, they get what they deserve. Or perhaps you like to read. You know, books? Who has time? Do you know the real reason social media is so popular? Because a 280-character tweet is the only thing parents have time to read start to finish.

However, there are some things you might be able to control. For example, pets. Eventually, your offspring will want pets. Maybe you can get away with a fish, and if you can, good for you. I'm a fan of pets, mainly because I like to see my kids pick up poop, given our own adventures in diapering. This is only fair. What I did not realize is that the pets would also need to be in the bathroom with me. I'm not a wealthy woman – I have what I need, and I certainly have enough. But my bathroom real estate is remarkably ill equipped to handle two dogs, three cats, two children, and whatever lizard/praying mantis/dung beetle happens to be in my son's hand. I neglected to ask for the Noah's Ark of bathrooms when house hunting. My mistake. One of our pets is part cattle dog, and I am his special person. Meaning he can't be more than two feet away from me without having an anxiety attack. Add to this fact that my kids often have people over, and you can see the problem.

If you are female, you've gotten well used to the lack of privacy by the time you have a child. The disappearing hospital gowns alone are excellent practice for the utter lack of privacy you'll experience as a parent. As a young woman I was offered a full-length fabric hospital gown when I disrobed at the doctors. That became a shorter fabric gown. Then back to full length, but it was paper. And now? Now it is a tiny paper vest, too flimsy to blow your nose on. I can only assume next time they'll hand me a cocktail napkin and call it a day.

Of course, the act of giving birth can give you great insight into what's to come. The utter lack of modesty about to invade your world. With my first child, there were oh, I don't know, nineteen people in the room? Lovely Hubby of course, and my doctor (eventually) and my nurse, and a nurse for the baby, and an assistant for that nurse, and an anesthesiologist for the epidural, and the nurse who came in to talk about the shift change, and the nurse who came in to get my doctor because the other pregnant woman was moving faster than I was, and the nurse who was there to change the wall paper, and then the fry cook and the waitress with my drink order... I've had smaller crowds on opening night. On this particular opening night, it didn't matter. Never mind that it was my vagina opening. Honestly. I'm a very modest person in real life. In writing yes, I'll give you an entire chapter on my vagina if need be but in person, very modest. Even a thousand years ago when I was acting – even when I was the least dressed character on stage, still modest. Although a theater dressing room is a good place to practice not caring who sees what. I once had a thirty-five second full costume change – top to bottom including shoes and earrings. Needless to say I walked from one side of backstage to the other while people undressed and re-dressed me. But there were always a ton of stagehands around and they were super helpful.

So, on some level, there is an audience for the birth of your child. I'm not talking about the filming and showing of the birth to the people who will pretend they enjoy watching your vagina stretch beyond comprehension; I'm talking about the actual number of people in the room.

I know people who set up cameras so they could watch the birth of their child while they did it.

Not me.

I had my eyes closed. I just wanted to feel everything that was happening. And when I opened my eyes, my daughter was looking straight into my eyes. And everyone else disappeared. I'm not sure how long we stayed like that, but eventually time started again. Mainly because I was so friggin' hungry I was going to kill someone if I didn't get a burger STAT.

Luckily none of it matters. Because in that crowd of thousands watching the birth of my first child, it was completely silent. And when she arrived and begin to squall and everyone relaxed, I heard a nurse say quietly:

"Every time, it gets me every time."

And that was the last time I was alone with my thoughts. Approximately 7:56 pm on a Tuesday night in 2006.

SHH... THE CHILDREN ARE TALKING

Growing up in the seventies we were on our own a lot, as you've likely gathered. Left to our own devices caused a lot of problems, but it also meant a lot of opportunities to just figure stuff out. And growing up Italian meant two things – food, and family. And food. The food was constant. And the family was constantly at top volume. Lovely Hubby and I have the full volume part down, and occasionally the food is decent. The family, well, as may be painfully evident by now, I did not do a lot of reading up before I had kids. My vague notion was that my children were born knowing everything they need to know, and that my husband and I most likely mess up that wisdom in profound ways each and every day. Having been parents for some time now we are trying to enjoy what we can and minimize the ill effects of our parenting.

What's the old joke? You can raise a child by the book, but you need a different book for every child. I didn't read them (lazy) but I did give the best parenting books on the market to my children. They chewed on the corners, built them into towers they knocked down, and occasionally ripped out pages. Possibly entire chapters. Could it be a coincidence that they didn't agree with prepping for college while in pre-school? Tough to say. Clearly they know something I don't... but what? I decided to observe my children for a few weeks, I mean really pay attention not just feed and water them out of service to this book and this is what I learned:

1. The toilet paper will reach from the master bath all the way to the back door of the kitchen.
2. The child lock isn't working if your toddler hands it to you.
3. A pasta box will fit on your hand, but not your head, so save yourself some frustration.
4. Yams make an excellent facial.
5. You can feed the dog by putting the food in the dish, near the dish, or all over the living room. Or just wait for her to jump into your lap in your highchair.
6. A skinned knee is no reason to slow down or change direction.
7. A little honesty goes a long way.
8. When in doubt, take a bath. When really in doubt, eat dinner in the bath.
9. If you learn a really good word, use it for everything. Example: Do you want a snack? Purple.
10. Playing with a baseball is fun until it hits you in the face. Likewise, it's fun to jump on the couch until you smack your face into the arm rest. Then it's slightly less fun but still better than going to bed.
11. Just because your split lip is gushing blood doesn't mean you can't enjoy an airplane going by overhead. Run as fast as you can at all times.
12. If you ate, played and pooped, it's perfectly reasonable to nap.
13. Putting things back in the box is never as fun or as easy as taking them out.
14. Wearing a tiara can really lift your day. The best way to eat noodles? With your hands. The longer the better.
15. Body parts really do make the best toys – belly buttons, feet,

ears, etc. They can be your body parts or someone else's, doesn't really matter. Next best is a good spoon.

16. Why *isn't* a pocketbook a book you fit in your pocket?
17. Naked. Try it.
18. Popcorn with cinnamon and sugar. Try it. Try it naked and get as much butter on yourself as possible.
19. Cats are faster than dogs to run away.
20. It's possible to cause two additional spills before the first one is cleaned up.
21. Smile at people, they smile back. If you keep smiling, they say hello. If you keep smiling, they ask your name, and maybe how old you are, and how you got to be such a happy boy. Just keep smiling. Soon you will have a crowd. Everyone will want to know why you are so smiley. Maybe toss a few lucky ones a high five or blow them a kiss. Have your stroller whisk you away from a job well done.
22. Just because you don't fit between the couch and the wall, doesn't mean you can't keep trying.
23. If it's there, climb it.
24. Every now and then, stop what you're doing and lie down on the floor, and check things out from that angle. If you're up to it, make a carpet angel (you know, like a snow angel, only on a carpet).
25. There is a magnetic attraction between toddlers and power cords. The strength of the attraction is in direct and inverse relationship to how far away a parent is.
26. Intention is everything. Which is why the dog lets the baby pull on her tongue.
27. You are living in the moment when the jack in the box surprises you every time.
28. Even Trade: The aggravation of losing things is balanced by the joy of not ever cleaning your room.
29. The common garden rake is an underestimated housecleaning tool.
30. What's better than having one flag to wave? Two. What's

better than two? Three. What's better than three? Four. What's better than four?

31. If you have the right age difference between your children, you need only buy one toy. The older child gets the toy. The younger child gets the box.
32. Now is the best time to sit and read a book together.
33. Meryl Streep has nothing on a toddler that doesn't want to nap. The depths of tragedy that are occurring right now in my house would rival any natural disaster, if everyone who survived that disaster was immediately diagnosed with stage four cancer of everything and Alzheimer's. I am certain to be arrested shortly for inducing this much misery into one very small person. If he doesn't fall asleep soon, I will have to flagellate myself for the mere suggestion of a nap- oh, good, he nodded off.
34. Farts are funny. They just are. They feel funny, and they make other people make funny faces when they smell them. So don't be such a snooty patootie about it.
35. Strollers are an excellent form of travel, allowing for maximum snack time, sleep time, and observation time.
36. Just because you say it's not a toy, doesn't mean I won't play with it.
37. You really need to get over yourself and not care what other people think, because: My good mood is in inverse proportion to (a) how far we are from home (b) how many snacks you remembered to pack (c) whether or not there are balloons. And most important (d) how embarrassed you would be if I started to Wail. Right. Now.
38. Sometimes no means yes if you ask 9,495,234,501,333,968 times.
39. Any mention of ice cream is a blood oath and will be remembered until fulfilled.
40. The TV is a babysitter. That is its only purpose. How else does dinner get made?
41. "Mom, I want you to do the things for me that I want you to

do, but not the things that I'm big enough to do myself, and I may change my mind at any moment as to what belongs in either category. Oh, and there's a third group, which is things I don't want anyone to do, ever. Good luck."

42. It has to be difficult to have someone else make all the decisions for you. Like having a personal assistant who doesn't listen to what you want.
43. If we aren't supposed to put our fingers in our nose, then why do they fit so perfectly?
44. There is always a reason to laugh.
45. There is a fourth form of matter which is neither solid, liquid nor gas and is currently in my toddlers' diaper.
46. It's possible to look at someone and know, "Mom, we're going to be best friends."
47. Just because it's below freezing doesn't mean a jacket is necessary. Or even a shirt.
48. Why is it the Sandman? Why can't it be the Sandgirl? Why is it Jack Frost? Why can't it be Jill Frost?
49. Exhaustion is no reason to take a nap. Go, go, go!
50. Why aren't *people* just *people*? Why are there white people and African American people and Indian people?
51. Also, if you say the word people a bunch of times in a row, it starts to sound really funny. People, people, people, people, people, people, people, people. See? Works if you type it too.
52. Paint is great, no matter what it ends up on. But glue is best for sticking hands together. Your own, or someone else's.
53. The space between the toilet and the wall is perfect for parking your tractor.
54. Vacation philosophy – Enjoy all of it. The shuttle from the parking lot is as much fun as the tram ride to the gate, which is as much fun as the plane ride which is as much fun as funny little bathroom on the plane, which is as much fun as the bus to the hotel, which is as much fun as the monorail to the amusement park, which is just as good as riding the elephant ride in the air.

55. You can actually step into a toilet.
56. Sometimes, when times are rough, if you just keep saying "no" long enough, whatever is bugging you will eventually go away.
57. "Me, me, me, me, me". It's OK to put yourself first. Particularly when cookies are at stake, but I suspect for other things as well.
58. Naked! Naked! Can't say enough about how great it is to be Naked!
59. If you master the business end of the spoon, it's time to try using the flat end.
60. If Mom says no juice, ask Dad. If Dad says no juice, ask your sister. If she says no, go back and take your mom by the hand and lead her out of the kitchen. Then get a box and climb up and get some juice.
61. Cute gets away with a lot. Cute with a dimple gets away with damn near everything.
62. Dessert is not a treat. Dessert is an iron clad promise, a legal and binding contract. Sweets are a birthright. See *ice cream* for details.
63. A snow day is nature's alarm clock.
64. Adults lack enthusiasm. It's unforgivable.
65. An apology is best when it comes unbidden.
66. Making a mess isn't making a mess. It's just playing. They aren't making a mess. They are making a ________.
67. My kids can't read my mind. This one was a shock let me tell you.
68. Cheer for what you want more of in the world– "go snow, go down, go go go, go snow!"
69. A lopsided heart card beats store bought any day.
70. My toddler needs his privacy. Even if he is sitting on a little potty buck naked in the middle of the hallway. If you're bored on your little trainer potty? Scoot it down the hall to someplace new and interesting while you wait for the pee to come.

71. Be clear: "please put your dish in the sink" does not indicate the velocity with which it should be hurled.
72. Sometimes it takes the entire softball team cooing over your baby brother to remind you how much you love him.
73. Time slows down for kids and speeds up for parents (and vice versa) in direct opposition.
74. Everyone just wants love, food, and a cozy place to nap.
75. A person who loves to read is never lonely.
76. Colored sugar (liquid, solid, or cotton candy) is a food group.
77. The "I love veggies" window may only be open very briefly. Take advantage.
78. If you don't want your kid to act like a movie star, don't act like a personal assistant.
79. Rain boots qualify as shoes, regardless of weather.
80. Toddlers wear pants so they can't get their diapers off.
81. Smothering yourself in paint is more fun than smothering paper in paint. Smothering someone else in paint is even better. The bathtub is the best place for all painting projects. Or the neighbor's house.
82. A screaming child, like a barking dog, is an effective way to avoid a conversation with a door-to-door salesperson.
83. For a person without children, a temper tantrum is a sign of bad parenting.
84. An effective way to wake a sleepy toddler is to accidentally smack their head on the hatchback door trying to get them into the hiking backpack carrier thing.
85. Sometimes not crying is scarier to witness than crying, as in, "Why isn't he crying after I accidentally smacked his head on the hatchback door trying to get him into the hiking backpack carrier thing?"
86. Ice cream. Is. Always. Welcome.
87. Any surface greater than ½ inch above the ground must be climbed. Repeatedly. Examples: A book, a chair, a tree, a vacuum.

88. Just because it's called a rocking horse doesn't mean you can't stand on it surfer style.
89. Snaggle tooth smiles are gorgeous.
90. Peeing outside feels funny.
91. Cleaning the house = discovery of forgotten toys = new mess = cleaning the house...
92. Salmon plus asparagus = best meal ever... wait two weeks... Salmon +asparagus = worst meal ever...wait for it...then Salmon + asparagus = best meal ever.
93. Beware the baby who realizes he can take off his own diaper.
94. Babies get everything. EVERYTHING (stamp foot and scowl for full effect).
95. Poop defies the laws of gravity. Poop is also the stickiest substance known to humankind. If it didn't smell so bad, it could probably have some fantastic uses.
96. If she says she can do it herself, she can do it. Her. Self.
97. Toilet paper right off the roll. It's not just for breakfast anymore. I have no idea what this refers to.
98. Boys who look straight at you are trying to flirt with you.
99. Need a wiggly tooth to come out? Put a pot on your head and dance around singing about milk.
100. A fabulously round belly (and belly button) is something to be proud of and should be shown immediately to anyone who asks.
101. Allowing a hot pink permanent marker in your house is an invitation to draw on your best carpet.
102. There's a very fine line between fighting and fun.
103. There's a very fine line between enough water for a bath and a tsunami in the bathroom.
104. Marker + paper = art. Marker + couch = controversial art
105. Confusion = applause for poop in the potty, but not on the floor.
106. Total conviction = a child denying they drew on the wall while holding the crayon. To the wall. And moving it. In a drawing fashion.

107. I can so pick up four balls at once. What do you think my chin is for?
108. Mom, just because I said your name 100 times does not mean I need you.
109. Math still sucks, but there are now thousands of new ways to do the same old math problem. With the same answer.
110. The best toys have neither batteries nor directions.
111. "Mom, if they don't want me to kick the seat in front of me, why do they place the airplane seats so close together?"
112. You can't sneeze out a bead once you shove it up your nose.
113. Outside is more fun than inside.
114. An angler fish has teeth in its throat. (What, you're saying you knew that?)
115. Need a quick disguise? Smear maple syrup all over your face, and say, 'ho ho ho I'm Santa Claus.' It doesn't matter if it's February. Everyone will be fooled.
116. Why can't you dip a stuffed monkey into your yogurt? No, really, why can't you dip a stuffed monkey into your yogurt?
117. Sing with me now...Climb every mountain... try every potty...
118. Options for popcorn (a) eat it (b) spread it out on the floor, and drive your cars over it (c) advanced players only: stuff as many pieces as possible in, under and around the wheels of your car. Then, try to figure out why your car won't roll.
119. Absolutely anything held up to your ear is a phone. Don't limit yourself to the standard toy version, or even that tired old banana. Poppycock. Use a napkin. A rock. Or a cat. Or my personal favorite, a jump rope. Just drag it along behind you in a completely unintentional reference to a telephone cord. No contract required.
120. It's hard to eat cereal with a fork. It's not impossible, but it's hard.
121. If you have trouble sleeping, practice being a chameleon that spies a caterpillar to eat. Shift your eyes quickly from side to

side, then suddenly; let them bug out as you lock in on the tasty caterpillar in front of you.

122. Sometimes you have to sit on the couch like a vegetable. Lie like broccoli. Particularly if the boogers coming out of your nose are the color of broccoli.
123. A bicycle may only have one seat, but that doesn't mean two people can't ride it. More importantly, one person can also ride two bicycles. Not well mind you, but it can be done.
124. The alarm button on the elevator is well within reach.
125. Correction to the earlier statement: Poop is not the stickiest substance in the known universe. Dried snot is the stickiest known substance in the known universe. For maximum effectiveness, smear it sideways across your cheek in an impossibly thin layer, covering your face from nostril to earlobe. It also has "magnetic" properties, attracting everything from dog hair to glitter to lint to very small gravel. Or perhaps that's kitty litter. Hard to say.
126. The more important it is to get out the door on time, the more fun it is to run away from your coat.
127. If you put enough gum on someone's chair, like, say, your mom's, she will stick to the chair, and then you don't ever have to go to bed. In theory.
128. Appropriate party behavior is to run around in circles as fast as you can, around and around and around and around, and then every now and then scream AAAAAAIIIIIIIEEEEEEEEEEEE!!!! And then collapse, sweating for a moment or two, and do it again.
129. Don't let the truth get in the way of playtime. Example: Deny that you have poop in your pants and need a diaper change. No one will know. When asked what the smell is, say "I'm fine." Alternatively, you can go in the corner and face the wall to do your business- no one will notice.
130. Bored? Say someone's name over and over and over and over and over and then pretend you've forgotten what you were going to say to them.

131. No really, think OUT of the box. This is the 8 year old teaching the 2 year old math,"Say 3 minus 2 equals 1." He replies, "3 minus 2 equals 1." "Good. What does 3 minus 2 equal?" "Chicken."
132. If you try to make me sit on the potty, I'm just going to run down the hall naked and my poop will end up in your shoe. Chill on the potty training.
133. Toddler morning coffee = staring out the front window at the garbage trucks and school buses going by.
134. A toy you haven't seen in a month or more is brand new. If it happens to be in the donate box, it is immediately your favorite toy ever. You can't live without it. You can't believe it's been withheld from you for so long. Something must be done to prevent this travesty – how could you possibly donate a toy that you begged to own months and then played with for seven minutes, and then left in the laundry hamper? Why do you even have to ask these questions?
135. Fireflies want to be free. Inside the house.
136. Live life like this: !!!!!!!!!

A SNEAK PREVIEW

CONVERSATION WITH A TWEEN

Today's special is brought to you by frustration and pride, the prevailing emotions of parents everywhere. And pee, the prevailing liquid on the bathroom floor. At least I hope it's pee.

"What did you do in school today?"

Silence

"Did you learn anything?"

"No."

"Did you talk about anything?"

"No."

"Was your teacher in class today?"

"Teachers? I don't know."

"Are the walls of the school still standing?"

"Huh?"

"Do you have homework?"

"No. Yeah. I don't know. What can I eat?"

"Whatever you want."

"Can you make me a ham and bacon sandwich with sliced tomatoes and just a little cheese sprinkled on top, oh, and pickles, but only if we have actual round ones not the long stinky ones and can you toast it please? And if we have Lemon Lime Super Slurpee then with sea salt chips and if not then regular chips and then I want Dr. Pepper but only if it's in a mini-can."

Pause

Pause

Pause

"Where are your shoes?"

A LAST WORD OF ADVICE

First, don't take parenting advice. Don't take it. "What?" you scream, "Why did I buy this book?" It's a barely hidden fact of the publishing industry that we often require readers to do the opposite of what we say. Example – every book on de-cluttering should begin with the phrase "don't buy this book, get it from the library." I feel like that would be the proper way to start that type of book. Now, I wish I could write that type of book, but we all know I can't because my house is so cluttered up with books on de-cluttering.

Let me re-phrase: Don't take anyone else's advice, except mine and yours. I assume you want my thoughts or you wouldn't be reading this. Or perhaps you're staying in a cabin or hotel I've been to and left copies of my book in, accidentally on purpose.

Allow me to revise: My rule is simply this: *I* do not take *unsolicited* parenting advice from anyone who was not directly involved in the making of my children. So, if you weren't in the room when they were born – not interested. Now if I ask for advice, that's different. I often joked that my siblings were my second set of parents. And in many ways, they were. My brother once convinced an entire dorm of men (it was a Catholic college) to ignore me when I visited for the entire weekend because I was only sixteen and he'd kill them if they spoke to me. That weekend did not go as I planned.

So, before we leave, here's some advice I took when I ignored my own advice about taking advice:

1. You are already making parenting decisions; right down to deciding whether or not you want to have children. There's really no zero to sixty involved in parenting. Just keep doing what you're doing.
2. Make the best decision you can based on the information you have. I know a couple who ripped out their brand new hardwood floor because of report on wood glue in cribs. That's fine, whatever makes you feel better, I'm just saying, every six months, every six weeks, every six minutes there is something new to be terrified of so pace yourself.
3. You cannot love your child too much. You simply cannot. There is no negative to this – love them, and love them, and love them.
4. Pick your battles. There is no such thing as a perfect child. That species does not exist.
5. And this from my parents, whose best advice was not directly about parenting possibly because I waited until my mid-thirties to have children, possibly because I never listened to them about anything in the past, possibly because they are wise and know that unsolicited advice. Grates. On. My. Nerves. Anyway, their advice for life is this, and I think it's brilliant: Get involved in your community. Wherever you live, volunteer; participate in making that community better in some way. This is excellent parenting advice. Think of everything that is rolled up in that simple statement –make the community better, care about something beyond your own front door, acknowledge that there are things that need changing in the world. Plus, it doesn't give you permission to

wait around for someone else to do it. You are responsible for making the world a better place for all the other humans living in it. Oh yes, I know, the response of some of you will be, yeah, but not everyone does that, so why should I? Well, that's really for you to answer. I'm just saying, that would not fly where I grew up.

NOTES

64. FIND YOUR PARENTING SPIRIT ANIMAL

1. The delightful BBC America special Animal Parents has actual scientific facts regarding these animal parenting skills. Assuming "science" and "fact" still mean anything at the time of publication.

ACKNOWLEDGMENTS

Too many thanks to thank to…

To my husband, who is my opposite in nearly every way and my perfect fit- we parent together remarkably well, I think, and it seems to be working out OK, and if it doesn't we'll just say it was the kids' fault. Mille grazii per tutti.

To my children, who made me a parent, you got your own chapter so seriously? Seriously, if I was able to express my love, gratitude and pride that I can call you my children, I'd be a much better writer. I simply cannot do you justice.

To my brother and sister, who were remarkably strict in parenting me and remarkably supportive at the same time, you are what I wish I could be as a parent.

And to my parents, who had to parent me, thank you for making me feel like the center of the universe, and for letting me push back so very hard, it told me that I had something worth saying.

To the doctor who didn't deliver me and the nurse who did. To the doctors who saved my life oh so many years later and the nurses and techs who made sure it stuck. To LB, the other member of the world's tiniest gang - thank you for being my constant sounding board for this and so many other important things in my life. To Bel, KNP and Brad for reading it when it was a pile of words and phrases.

To the many, many, many women who have shown me what it is to be a good person and a good mom. Not that I'm either of those, but I appreciate the examples you set. To Khea, Meredith, and Meg whose advice or anecdotes worked their way into these pages. To Annie and Erin and Liam three of my favorite humans.

To Julie, Gina, Debbie, Cherie, Michelle, Amy, Christian, AnnMarie, and Kathleen.

Finally, to the readers of #bookstagram, the book club of my dreams.

THANK YOU

Dear Reader,

Thank you for reading *Birth and Other Surprises,* without you I am not an author, I'm just a collector of words and phrases on a page. I hope this book helped you realize what a terrific parent you are. It's true, I've heard great things. Also I read your diary.

Would you be so kind as to review it? It doesn't have to be lengthy to have an impact. True story - the definitions in this book were inspired by an online reader's review. As we say in theater, if you liked it, tell your friends, if you didn't, tell your enemies.

There are a lot of places to review, including Amazon, GoodReads, ReadersFavorite - you can even send me your review directly at KDBassoWrites@gmail.com. No joke. I read them. I look forward to hearing from you, and have a clot free day.

kdb

ABOUT THE AUTHOR

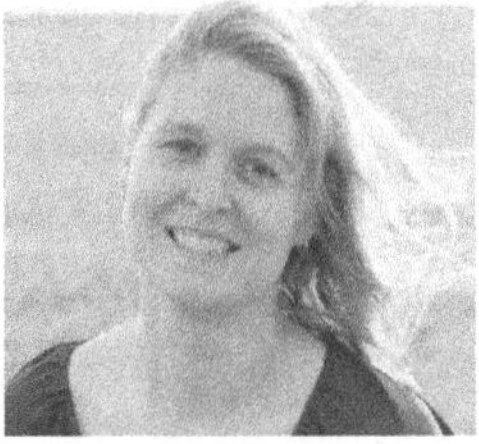

Kimberly Davis Basso is an author, playwright and speaker with many shiny stickers for her books, including nominations for INDIES Book of the Year in Humor from Foreword Reviews and Life Stories Book of the Year Finalist from Writer's Digest. Kimberly is a stroke survivor, and will speak with any group, anywhere about stroke awareness and how your children can help you in a medical emergency - yours.

Kimberly resides in a tiny cottage in California with Lovely Hubby, two smaller humans she helped create, two dogs and three cats. She invites you to get in touch in whatever method you prefer. She can't promise the cats won't eat a carrier pigeon but she'd love to see the Pony Express come through. She is on Twitter and Insta @KDBWrites and you can always find her via her website, www.KimberlyDavisBasso.com.

facebook.com/KDBwrites
twitter.com/kdbwrites
instagram.com/kdbwrites

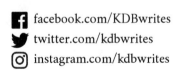

ALSO BY KIMBERLY DAVIS BASSO

I'm a Little Brain Dead

The Bride

Hollow

CPSIA information can be obtained
at www.ICGtesting.com
Printed in the USA
LVHW020716250220
648116LV00005B/863

9 781734 552300